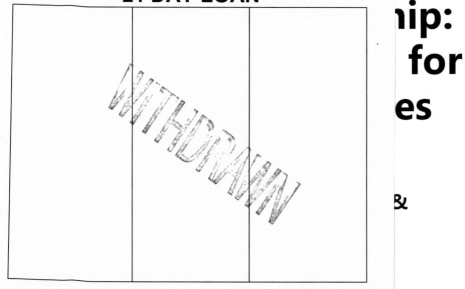

ⅰ|ip:
for
es

&

7.doc   v:18052005   geggro

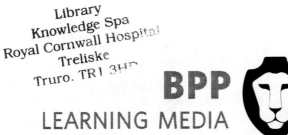

First edition November 2011

ISBN 9781 4453 7957 9
e-ISBN 9781 4453 8586 0

British Library Cataloguing-in-Publication Data
A catalogue record for this book is available from
the British Library

Published by
BPP Learning Media Ltd
BPP House, Aldine Place
London W12 8AA

www.bpp.com/health

Typeset by Replika Press Pvt Ltd, India
Printed in the United Kingdom

Your learning materials, published by BPP
Learning Media Ltd, are printed on paper
sourced from sustainable, managed forests.

BPP
LEARNING MEDIA

Contents

Contents

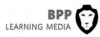

Contents

Contents

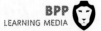

About the Publisher

BPP Learning Media is dedicated to supporting aspiring professionals with top quality learning material. BPP Learning Media's commitment to success is shown by our record of quality, innovation and market leadership in paper-based and e-learning materials. BPP Learning Media's study materials are written by professionally-qualified specialists who know from personal experience the importance of top quality materials for success.

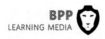

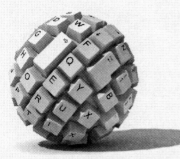

Free Companion Material

Readers can access all of the references in this book (to other books, PubMed citations and web links) in a convenient 'medical leadership references' document for free online.

To access the above companion material please visit **www.bpp.com/freehealthresources**

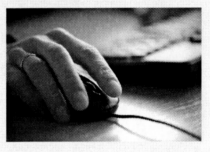

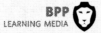

About the Authors

Peter Spurgeon

Peter Spurgeon is currently Director of the Institute for Clinical Leadership at the University of Warwick Medical School. He has previously been Director of the Health Services Management Centre, University of Birmingham, and for the past four years has been seconded to the Institute for Innovation and Improvement and the Academy of Medical Royal Colleges as Project Director of the Enhancing Engagement in Medical Leadership programme. He has worked on many overseas assignments and holds chairs in Italy and Australia.

Bob Klaber

Bob Klaber is a Consultant Paediatrician at Imperial College Healthcare NHS Trust and has trained as a medical educationalist. He continues to be involved in leading educational initiatives and educational research projects as well as having an active role as a clinical and educational supervisor. He has a particular interest in the development of leadership and management skills in doctors and other healthcare professionals, and worked as a medical advisor with the project team that developed the Medical Leadership Competency Framework. Driven by a desire to facilitate junior doctors in developing these skills within a work-based setting, he has both led and supported a number of different leadership development schemes and initiatives within the UK, and established the paired-learning pilot for managers and clinicians in London in 2010, which is described in the final chapter of this book.

Contributors

Chapter 7
Francesca Cleugh

Chapter 8
Amna Suliman & Oliver Warren

Chapter 9
David Griffiths

Chapter 10
Katie de Wit

Chapter 11
Lizzie Smith

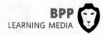

Acknowledgements

I would like to thank all colleagues in the Enhancing Engagement in Medical Leadership project for their work in creating the source material (John Clark, Penny Lewis, Isobel Down, Kirsten Armit, Marijka Trickett and Tracy Lonetto). Particular thanks goes to Emma Darbey for help in producing the manuscript.

Peter Spurgeon
November 2011

It has been a fantastic combination of fun and challenge in writing this book, but none of it would have happened without the amazing support of my wife Jo, and my three wonderful children, who are slowly coming to terms with the idea of a book that has no dragons, fairies nor princesses in it.

I want to say a huge thank you to Peter for all of his help in driving this project forward, and to Fran (Paediatric EM SpR), David (GP), Oliver (Surgical SpR), Amna (Surgical Trainee), Katie (Medical Student) and Lizzie (NHS Manager) for their brilliant work in writing / co-writing their chapters. The fact that such outstanding and committed people, who are very much on the frontline of clinical work, gave up so much time to contribute has given the book real life and credibility, and I very much hope that will shine through for you as a reader.

Much of the inspiration for the ideas in the book has come from time spent with my very medical family, and the wonderful colleagues who I have been lucky enough to work with over the years. I am immensely grateful for their support and direction. It has been a real privilege to write about a subject that I passionately believe has a vastly important role in improving patient care.

Finally I would like to thank Matt, Sabrina, Ruth and the team at BPP Learning Media for all of their hard work in getting this book published.

Bob Klaber
November 2011

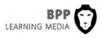

Images

The authors and BPP Learning Media are grateful for the NHS Institute for Innovation and Improvement and the Academy of Medical Royal Colleges for their kind permission to reproduce the Medical Leadership Competency Framework logos and figures. These appear in the following sections:

- Figure 2.1 and Figure 2.2 in Chapter 2
- Regularly throughout Chapters 4–10
- Fly pages for Chapters 1–11

These images are © 2010 NHS Institute for Innovation and Improvement and Academy of Medical Royal Colleges. All rights reserved.

References

References are given in full at the end of each chapter.

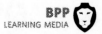

Foreword by Professor Parveen Kumar CBE

The challenges currently facing healthcare systems across the world are immense and made more taxing in the climate of a global recession. Financial constraints have to be balanced against the steeply rising costs of modern technology, new innovative medicines and rising patient and public expectations. The modern patient is now a 'medical expert' with knowledge gleaned from the countless 'doctor' programmes on the television and easy internet access. They also have little time in their busy lives to seek medical opinion and expect instant medical care with the most modern technological advances. So delivering the best possible care to our patients and the public is becoming an even more complex and daunting issue.

On top of all this, the profession is itself is undergoing massive changes in education and in training, as well as the changing roles of doctors, nurses and other healthcare professionals. How should we educate our future doctors to make them fit for their future working lives? How should young trainees be taught in order to accommodate the European Working Time Directive? What about the training for nurses and other healthcare professionals? What is the most cost-effective method to train in the context of a shorter time to study and more intensive workload without compromising patient care? All these require difficult and complex decisions which will involve changes in service across a multidisciplinary arena and need to be managed properly.

The medical profession has been slow to take on the challenge of medical management and leadership and has, in the past, been content to run their clinical and academic teams in strictly controlled silos. This is now not only inappropriate but a huge barrier for multidisciplinary teams to work together in the pursuance of giving good medical care to patients. We need to look beyond our local environments and cross the boundaries of disciplines, careers and our own selfish enterprise.

So where does this leave us? 'You are a born leader' is a phrase often used to imply leadership qualities in a person, but I wonder whether it has the same resonance nowadays. No doubt some people might have the inherited attributes for a leadership role but, leadership nowadays is more than just an art: it has become a science as well. It has to be learned within the context of various aspects and levels of leading and managing.

This book forms the basis for approaching many of the above daunting issues. It teases out various problems and offers practical advice based on real life examples from our daily working practice. It discusses the interrelationships between management and leadership and goes on to consider leadership learning in the various hospital and primary care environments. I was particularly interested in the advice for leadership learning as an undergraduate. I have always advocated an early introduction to leadership and management in the undergraduate curriculum.

The book is very readable, well set out and offers practical advice in an engaging way! There is also free companion material online with references and web links which will be very useful for a hard-pressed learner. The book is a 'must' for every healthcare worker, and not just for the 'born leader', as we all have a role in leadership and management... whether we like it or not!

Professor Parveen J Kumar
CBE MD FRCP FRCPE FRCPath
Professor of Medicine and Education
Bart's and the London School of Medicine and Dentistry,
Queen Mary University of London
President of the Royal Society of Medicine
Co-author of Kumar and Clark's *Clinical Medicine*

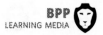

Forewords by Junior Doctors

A unique position of being a junior doctor is that you offer a new perspective on the healthcare system. It constantly demands innovation from us, yet our ability to do so can feel constrained by hierarchy and our relative inexperience. Though audits are encouraged, they can feel little more than a box-ticking exercise. This book is an inspiration because it enthuses you to take charge. Moreover, the case studies make it a practical guide on how to harness that box-fresh enthusiasm of being newly qualified into taking a lead in changing the way we work and improving our patients' care.

Dr Arnoupe Jhass
Foundation Year 1 Doctor
Poole General Hospital, UK

I once heard a senior colleague of Dr Klaber's refer to him as 'a monumental force knocking down organisational barriers... somewhat scary at times.' A fellow F2 doctor described him as 'so approachable and supportive, surely that's the way all consultants should be?!' Having worked with him in both clinical and academic environments, I have been inspired by his ability to somehow find creative and effective solutions to the perennial problems most of us learn to surrender to.

This book is an insight into this ingenious approach to the practical aspects of healthcare. Providing clear conceptual frameworks and relevant examples, the authors demonstrate how we can improve our work in a 'big picture', team-building manner, rather than struggling to navigate through the healthcare system as lone soldiers. It inspires us to act rather than complain, aiming not just for the production of great leaders, but also for a shift in culture in the NHS.

Dr Sabena Mughal
Foundation Year 2 Doctor
Ealing Hospital, London, UK

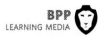

As doctors in training we have a unique role in the healthcare service, making key decisions about patient care and negotiating an often illogical system. As we develop our clinical practice and knowledge, we also need to develop the self-awareness, teamwork skills and systems understanding to enable us to give our patients the best possible care. We have all experienced the frustration of knowing what clinical care our patients need yet being unable to provide it, due to inefficient systems and poor communication.

This book provides down-to-earth, practical advice about how we can develop our leadership skills to address such problems. It recognises that doctors in training have multiple demands on their time and so focuses on the learning opportunities that exist in our clinical work. Rather than teaching 'leadership' as an abstract add-on to training, the authors use practical examples and exercises to embed the learning in our daily practice and help us see 'leadership' as meaningful and relevant to our roles. These are skills that will help us in our future roles as consultants and GPs but, just as importantly, will improve our practice right now at the start of our careers.

Dr Alice Roueché
Paediatric Specialist Registrar
London Deanery, UK

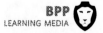

Chapter 1

Introduction

Peter Spurgeon

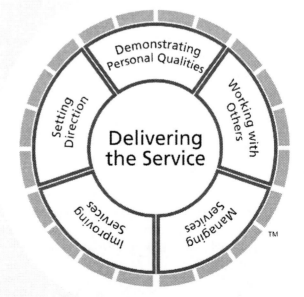

Introduction

 ### *Chapter overview*

This chapter provides:

- An outline of the origins and background to the widespread demand for enhanced medical leadership
- A rationale for the current focus on developing medical leadership
- A framework for using this book, from early chapters which offer a conceptual background to those offering practical learning opportunities within meaningful patient contexts

---

Background to the emergence and value of medical leadership

The concept of leadership is very fashionable, with the the search engine Google recording 122 million references, over 35 million of which relate to the public sector. It is not intended that busy professionals set off to review this vast set of material, so a very selective review will be presented here instead. This brief overview will seek to understand why leadership is such a popular concept both for researchers and practitioners and why it is so important in all stages of the medical career pathway.

The challenges facing the health system, in the UK and globally, are well rehearsed and indeed are the preface to the majority of policy and reform documents. Briefly, the major pressures on Western health systems can be outlined as:

- New patterns of disease, with an emphasis on chronic and multiple conditions
- New techniques, technology and drugs placing a financial burden upon the total health budget, and in many instances changing the pattern of healthcare delivery
- Heightened expectations from patients and carers emanating from a more educated population and the pre-eminent role afforded the consumer (patient and carer) in modern society

- An aging population with increasingly complex conditions exacerbated by complex cultural and ethnic needs
- A spotlight on issues of patient safety following high profile problems – in particular UK services (ie Bristol Heart Surgery; Mid-Staffordshire NHS Foundation Trust) and similar problems around the world

It is in response to this somewhat daunting list of pressures that leadership is seen as a solution. This can be observed in many sectors where inquiries or investigations into major incidents often report 'a failure of leadership' as a cause. This conclusion, and the complex and vast agenda in which it is set, raises questions about how leadership issues can be addressed. In the interest of balance, it should be said that such a list of pressures can often be presented as the basis for major reform, inadvertently or conveniently omitting other information such as: the highest level of reported satisfaction with the UK NHS; the UK health system ranking second out of seven countries by the most recent Commonwealth Fund assessment; and on specific dimensions of efficiency and effectiveness of care ranked first. It is not all doom and gloom. However, there is still a significant challenge in maintaining and improving health systems in the UK, especially in the light of required cost-saving targets of some £20 billion. Medical leadership will be a critical element in this.

Medical leadership: history and context

The term 'leadership' is itself subject to hundreds, if not thousands, of definitions. It is a complex concept, multifaceted, influenced by the setting in which it occurs and elusive – so much so that many authors opt out of providing a definition, leaving the reader to create their own broad sense of what is meant. There is some merit in this; because it is such a broad, encompassing term, individuals inevitably bring a sense of meaning and interpretation (albeit often stereotypical) to the term. As a simplified but operational approach, the definition used here is: *leadership is a process of influence whereby those subject to it are inspired, motivated or become willing to undertake the tasks necessary to achieve an agreed goal.*

Some would then argue that even if a working definition of leadership can be agreed, is it the same as clinical leadership ie is this distinct and different? Some might argue that clinical leadership is just a description of any individual in a clinical role who exercises leadership; others suggest that it is leadership by clinicians for clinicians. The latter would seem a dangerously narrow formulation, almost by definition excluding other areas of management or leadership activity. This is not the concept of medical leadership advocated here; we are discussing the skills of leadership directed by a person (clinician or not) to an area of activity that could secure improved patient care. Such leadership enactment would almost inevitably impact upon individuals other than clinicians alone.

Before proceeding, it is important that the issue so many commentators skirt around is addressed head on: is clinical leadership an all-embracing term covering all clinical professions, or is it confined to medical leadership?

Clinical leadership vs medical leadership

Most authors use the inclusive term *clinical leadership* and this certainly acknowledges the importance of teamwork in the delivery of modern healthcare. However, authors will equally use the term *clinical leadership* but then talk about doctors, and so they are really talking about *medical leadership*. A typical example of this would be found in Edmonstone who, when discussing clinical leadership programmes, quotes Nolan's survey of medical directors. This survey found that 90% of respondents felt there was no proper career structure to encourage medical staff to become clinical leaders, while 80% suggested that this role was not an attractive career option for doctors. The implication that leadership is an appropriate career route for nurses and other healthcare professionals was clear. Hence the confusion continues. To use the term *medical leadership* in no way diminishes the role and contribution of all other health professionals, but acknowledges a difference in education, training and – crucially – accountability.

The health sector is frequently directed to the aviation industry as a role model; the analogy with the crew (team) of an aircraft may be quite telling. Although operating as a team, the roles are occasionally different and not interchangeable. This is quite a subtle and contentious point in healthcare, as there is probably more role substitution and skill overlap in roles such as nurse practitioner. By advocating *medical leadership* as distinct from *clinical leadership*, it is not implied that the doctor is always the leader, and/or a better leader, in all circumstances. This is far from the case. However, what *is* suggested is that when leadership is exercised within a team, the professional identity, training and perspective of an individual is part of how this leadership role is enacted.

As a final pragmatic point, if the term 'clinical' was used, it would be necessary to continually point out throughout the book that the medical undergraduate course is of a different length and pattern to other clinicians, and that junior doctor roles are found in only one professional group and that it is this group which is moving to annual revalidation. For these and associated issues, such as power and influence as a professional group, the term *medical leadership* is used throughout. Please see Spurgeon, Clark and Ham for more discussion of this issue (reference at end of chapter).

A contextual framework to this book

The need for medical leadership is widely recognised on an international basis. Policy makers and the most senior NHS leaders are strong advocates. Why is this and is this a new development?

Taking a position that pre-dates the inception of the NHS, it seems that doctors, whether as individual practitioners or in early hospitals, were seen as leaders simply because of their training and expertise. Even after the NHS was formed and more doctors and other professionals were grouped together, each speciality and consultant exercised a form of leadership through the concept of clinical freedom and autonomy. Until relatively recently, doctors were not employed by the hospital in which they worked; local regional authorities held the contracts instead. This distinction reinforced the notion that as a profession, doctors sat outside the rest of the staff and were not a part of a managed community. The administrative structures grew up to support medical staff and the administrators, in turn – like most other staff – were seen as subsidiary to medicine as the lead profession.

The growth of managerialism

Certain key developments have shaped the current situation and brought about the requirement for the development of medical leadership. The first was the substantial growth of managerialism throughout the 1980s and 1990s. This process created a cadre of highly trained and very able managers who sought to progress from administrators to managers. *The Griffith Report* reinforced this movement. From a private sector perspective, Griffith advocated greater personal accountability and saw a need for doctors, as the key resource allocators, to work within the managed system. Even if conceptually valid, it was a recipe that failed to recognise historical positions. It led to a series of initiatives to contain spending and, as a matter of course, restrain the freedom of doctors to practise as they saw fit. The seeds of the oft-cited antagonism between doctors and managers can be found here. The scepticism of many doctors about the management process was established in these decades.

The second key point was post-2000, when a New Labour government rightly restored and enhanced funding to an under-resourced health service. The expectation was one of rapid improvement in process and outcome. Much of the extra funding resulted in more staff and salary increases. This was necessary but difficult to integrate with the desired productivity gains. The government's response was to set targets and direct the service centrally. Many doctors resented this and argued that they had not been consulted, and that many of the targets did not reflect clinical priorities. This may well have been true, but few would disagree that the targets achieved improvements in waiting times (in Emergency Departments) and waiting lists for elective procedures. It was in effect an uneasy stand-off, with the government frustrated by the failure of the service to roll out innovations and improvements as quickly as politicians wanted, while medical professionals, somewhat alienated and disaffected, were seen as the main, and most powerful, obstacle to rapid change.

By the mid 2000s it was clear that this position had to change if improvements were to be made, as desired and promised by governments. The situation moved from berating the profession because it would not change, to recognising that only if there was good medical leadership was it likely that the profession would

BPP
LEARNING MEDIA

develop a more positive perspective, enabling the required service improvements to be realised. It was in this way that medical leadership became a dominant theme.

The development of medical leadership

The rest of this book presents the response to the advocated position relating to medical leadership, together with an account of how this was achieved (Chapter 2), and some exploration in Chapter 3 of the relationship between management and leadership.

Following on from this conceptual overview, Chapters 4–11 provide several practical examples of how learners and educators can acquire leadership skills. The approach taken emphasises learning in a meaningful context – for example, on a hospital ward, in the operating theatre or in primary care. Some books have described leadership skills as items to be learnt or acquired with the belief (and hope) that the learner will be able to make the transition to application in a real-life setting. The overarching philosophy here is that the skills of leadership are integral to, and will improve, the practice of medicine, and are therefore better taught and acquired in realistic settings. Chapter 11 recognises that while everyone is a learner throughout their career, further benefit can be gained from guidance and support (in this instance form tutors and educational supervisors). These chapters provide a wide range of learning scenarios and exercises so that each reader can acquire skills a) in a practical context and b) that are of maximum direct relevance to the reader's present situation.

References

Davis K, Schoen C and Stremikis K. (2010) *Mirror, Mirror on the Wall: How the Performance of the US Health Care System Compares Internationally.* [Online] Available at www.commonwealthfund.org/content/publications/fund-reports/2010/jun/mirror-mirror-update.aspx?page=all [Accessed 17/10/11].

Edmonstone J ed. (2005) What is Clinical Leadership Development? In *Clinical Leadership: A Book of Readings.* Chichester: Kingsham Press. pp. 16–19.

Edmonstone J. Clinical Leadership: The Elephant in the Room. *International Journal of Health Planning and Management* 2009; 24: 290–305.

Hartley J and Benington J. (2010) *Leadership for Healthcare.* Bristol, UK: The Policy Press.

Ipsos MORI (2010) *Political and social trends.* [Online] Available at www.ipsos-mori.com/researchspecialisms/socialresearch/specareas/politics/trends.aspx [Accessed 17/10/11].

Malby B. Clinical Leadership. *Adv Pract Nursing* 1998; Q4 (3): 40–43.

Nolan A. Structural Instability. *Health Service Journal* 2006 (4 May).

Spurgeon P, Clark J and Ham C. (2011) *Medical Leadership: From the Dark Side to Centre Stage.* Oxford: Radcliffe Press.

Stanton E and Chapman C. (2010) Teamworking and clinical leadership. In Stanton E, Lemer C and Montford J eds. *Clinical Leadership: Bridging the Divide.* London: Quay Books.

The Department of Health and Social Security (DHSS) (1983) *NHS Management inquiry: The Griffith Report.* London: DHSS.

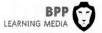

Chapter 2

The Medical Leadership Competency Framework

Peter Spurgeon

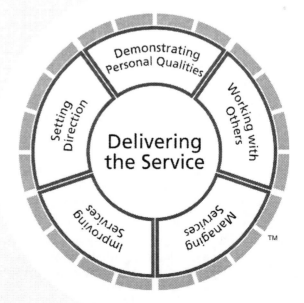

The Medical Leadership Competency Framework

 ## Chapter overview

This chapter provides:

- A background to the emergence of the Medical Leadership Competency Framework (MLCF)
- A review of the development of the MLCF and its embedding into the medical profession
- Information on further developments, built on the success of the MLCF

Introduction

As discussed in the previous chapter, there was a strong desire to enhance the engagement of doctors in the process of service change and improvement at the beginning of the 21st century. Implicit in this thinking was a recognition that doctors were not as well equipped as they might be to undertake (and lead) service change, nor were they, as a profession, always positively motivated to do so. Of course, by this time, a number of doctors had taken on leadership roles in their organisations with the British Association of Medical Managers (BAMM) co-ordinating much of the training and development for this group. Nonetheless, the numbers involved were relatively small. Medical leaders were a limited sub-set of the profession: not always particularly enthusiastic about the role, often quite transitional in terms of the time in post and still a slightly alienated, non-mainstream part of the profession. The challenge then was two-fold:

- How could the majority (not the minority) of doctors acquire the requisite management and leadership skills to play a full role in promoting service improvement?
- How could the culture surrounding medical managers and leaders be changed to support involvement in wider, non-clinical aspects of organisational performance, and therefore transform it into a natural and normal part of the medical role?

At the same time, there was increasing recognition from the medical professional, regulatory and educational bodies that the complexity of modern healthcare systems, coupled with the rapidity of change, required a more general examination of the adequacy of the current medical educational system. The previous individually-based clinical speciality curriculum was gradually moving to a broader competency-based model; the development of management and leadership skills had become a further component in this process.

Competency frameworks

Wass and Van der Vleuton define competency in the clinical context as *'the ability to handle a complex professional task by integrating the relevant cognitive, psychomotor and affective skills'* (2009). More broadly, and taking an organisational perspective, Lucia and Lepsinger suggest that competences can be defined as the knowledge, skills and attitudes that:

1.   Affect a major part of one's job (role or responsibility)
2.   Correlate with performance on the job
3.   Are measured against well-adapted standards
4.   Are improved by training and development

The competency-based approach has some clear benefits in describing what a competent professional (ie a doctor) is expected to be able to do in order to practise successfully in a particular context. Additionally, describing the knowledge, skills and attitudes involved in each competency facilitates both the design of curricula and the assessment process. In 2002, the first competency-based curricula were published by the three Royal Colleges of Physicians in the UK (Joint Committee for Higher Medical Training), representing a restructuring of training and assessment for specialist registrars.

In the context of management and leadership, a number of frameworks were emerging to address the need to describe what training content should be provided. The General Medical Council (GMC) published *Management for Doctors* and BAMM developed its own model, *A Syllabus for Doctors in Leadership and Management Positions in Healthcare*. Both of these frameworks were particularly oriented to medical leaders at a senior level and so, as mentioned

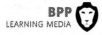

earlier, were aimed at supporting that relatively small group of doctors who had moved into medical leadership roles.

International competency frameworks

Elsewhere, the Royal College of Physicians and Surgeons of Canada developed the CanMEDS Roles Framework, with related competencies. This included quite a high level description of a set of roles – Professional, Communicator, Collaborator, Manager, Health Advocate and Scholar – which together combine to give 'The Medical Expert'. The Board of the National Union of Consultants in the Danish Medical Association also developed a model of leadership with five core competences:

- Personal leadership
- Leadership in a political context
- Leading quality
- Leading change
- Leading professionals

In the USA, McKenna et al. (2004, p. 348) highlighted more competences for physician leaders:

- Interpersonal and communication skills
- Professional ethics and social responsibility
- Continuous learning and improvement
- Ability to build coalitions and support for change
- Clinical excellence
- Ability to convey a clear compelling vision
- System-based decision-making/problem solving
- Ability to address needs of multiple stakeholders
- Financial acumen and resource management

Incidentally, the latter set is said to be in rank order. It is interesting to note the location of clinical excellence and financial acumen, which are often put forward as the basis of clinical leadership.

As you can see, there was quite an impetus at the time to define the additional areas of competence in management and leadership that were needed to ensure doctors could fulfil their role, both as clinical expert (the baseline) and to contribute to the running of the organisation. It is also clear that there is some overlap in the language and terms used and therefore suggests some degree of consensus. However, most of the frameworks described were still aimed at existing medical leaders and did not address the development pathway of medical education. Hence, they were not really addressing the second challenge mentioned earlier, of creating a new culture where these skills can be acquired and used as a normal part of the medical role.

The Medical Leadership Competency Framework (MLCF)

In the UK there was strong support for a systematic and coherent approach to the development of leadership skills across the key stages of the medical career. For example, the Royal College of Physicians produced a report, *Doctors in Society: Medical Professionalism in a Changing World*, where they argued:

> *The complementary skills of leadership and 'followership' need to be carefully documented and incorporated into a doctor's training to support professionalism. These skills argue strongly for managerial competence among doctors.*

(2005)

The NHS Institute for Innovation and Improvement and the Academy of Royal Medical Colleges jointly commissioned a project, Enhancing Engagement in Medical Leadership (EEML). This began in 2005 and was completed in March 2010. The EEML team consisted of senior NHS managers, medical advisors and academic advisors with access to other sources of information. The EEML is regarded as an extremely successful project, both in the nature of its process and outcome. A number of key factors contributed to this success, notably the thorough assessment of the relevant literature, wide-scale consultation (both before and during the conduct of the project), and incremental pilot testing. This allowed for the involvement of various stakeholder groups and the incorporation of their feedback into the emerging material. The project tasks included:

1. Reviewing the literature on medical leadership and engagement

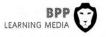

2. Reviewing the existing competency frameworks in the UK and internationally
3. Establishing a baseline of current activities and provision relating to leadership in medical training
4. Setting up several reference groups to advise the project team. These included senior medical staff, junior doctors, medical students, NHS managers and patient groups.
5. Consulting and establishing positive working relationships with a large number of key medical bodies (GMC, Medical Schools Council, British Medical Association, Royal Colleges etc.)

The overall aim of the project was to *'create a culture where doctors seek to be more engaged in management and leadership of health services, and non-medical leaders genuinely seek to improve services for patients'*. The critical output in this context was the development of the Medical Leadership Competency Framework (MLCF) which sought to *'define and describe the competences doctors need to become more actively involved in the planning, delivery and transformation of health services as a normal part of their role as doctors'*. The basic model of the MLCF is presented below:

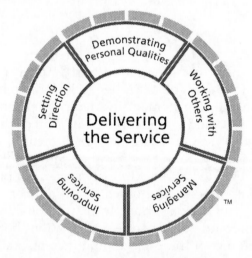

Figure 2.1 The Medical Leadership Competency Framework (MLCF)
Image © 2010 NHS Institute and AoMRC

The MLCF consists of five domains, with four elements in each domain; each of these is then divided into four competency outcomes.

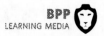

A listing of the domains and elements is given in Table 2.1 and a full description with learning suggestions is available on the NHS Institute website (www.institute.nhs.uk). Chapters 4–11 describe how doctors can acquire and develop these skills.

Domain
1. **Developing Personal Qualities** • Developing self awareness • Managing yourself • Continuing personal development • Acting with integrity
2. **Working with Others** • Developing networks • Building and maintaining relationships • Encouraging contribution • Working within teams
3. **Managing Services** • Planning • Managing recourses • Managing people • Managing performance
4. **Improving Services** • Ensuring patient safety • Critically evaluating • Encouraging improvement and innovation • Facilitating transformation
5. **Setting Direction** • Identifying the contexts for change • Applying knowledge and evidence • Making decisions • Evaluating impact

Table 2.1 The MLCF domains

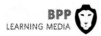

The development of the MLCF

The framework was extensively tested at every level and incorporates feedback from relevant groups. It is revised and updated annually to ensure the content is relevant and current.

The MLCF was designed to be relevant to all stages of the medical career pathway: undergraduate, postgraduate etc, as well as to the first revalidation following Certificate of Specialist Training. It therefore provides a cumulative map of relevant skills that can be acquired over time and to the appropriate level of development. For example, at undergraduate level it is unlikely that a student would be heavily involved in the fifth and most strategic domain, *Setting Direction*. However, working in teams and collaborating with others is an important part of learning to be a doctor and these skills can be introduced through situations relevant to the undergraduate.

The diagram below gives a very general sense of where particular aspects of the MLCF might be acquired across the medical career path. It must be emphasised though that potentially the whole framework is relevant at all times; the shading is simply indicative of emphasis and how likely situations will arise to offer learning opportunities.

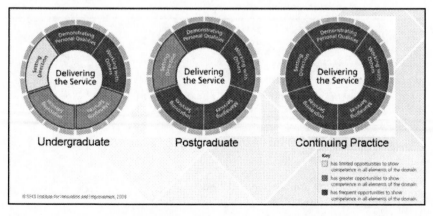

Figure 2.2 The MLCF across the medical career pathway (second edition).
Image © 2010 NHS Institute and AoMRC

The intention in developing the MLCF was to provide the content for training and development of doctors in management and

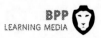

leadership. The progressive, cumulative nature of acquisition is also intended to provide a platform whereby skills in leadership would be acquired when relevant, but would gradually build to a good solid level of competence. This aspect in particular addresses the cultural issue of trying to ensure that all doctors acquire this essential grounding, so that when they take on specific leadership roles, eg clinical director, they have the background to move smoothly and competently into the role. The challenges posed by tasks associated with the role should also no longer feel alien, because they have been an integral part of the normal and natural development of the medical role. This was the intention and aspiration of the EEML project team.

Where are we now?

The development of the MLCF was the beginning of the process. To meet the more general goals of the project, it was essential that the MLCF became embedded into the training processes and therefore evolved as the consistent and universal basis for leadership development in the profession.

There were some absolutely crucial stages in the process of embedding. Of particular note, in the GMC's revised version of *Tomorrow's Doctors* (2009), the MLCF was cross-referenced as the basis for leadership training. Just as *Tomorrow's Doctors* is the document that prescribes the coverage and content of medical education in all medical schools in the UK, the MLCF became a required component of undergraduate training. Because each medical school has autonomy in the precise context of its curriculum, the extent of the leadership training is still evolving. However, a recent survey confirmed that the majority of medical schools have now begun integrating it into the curriculum. The GMC review-visits will further reinforce the requirement to reflect leadership in the undergraduate curriculum.

Leadership training at undergraduate level

At this stage of the project, the GMC was responsible for undergraduate education while a separate body, the Postgraduate Medical Education and Training Board (PMETB), was responsible for postgraduate education. In 2009, PMETB reviewed the MLCF, now translated as a curriculum, and agreed to ask all specialties to integrate the framework into their clinical curriculum so that it would become the basis of leadership training at postgraduate level. These were two vital markers in the embedding process and established the MLCF as the core leadership training content for doctors at undergraduate and postgraduate level. Currently, discussions with the GMC continue regarding the inclusion of MLCF in the review of *Good Medical Practice*. If secured, this would see the MLCF as the basis for a significant part of the medical career (it has always been acknowledged that in certain designated medical leadership roles, further training would be required, and may be specific to certain posts).

Leadership training at postgraduate level

Just as embedding at undergraduate level is a core strand, so too, and perhaps more so, is a parallel process at postgraduate level. Each Medical College now has a curriculum incorporating the MLCF; the responsibility for ensuring coverage of the MLCF and sufficient opportunities for trainees to develop their leadership competence falls to the Postgraduate Deaneries in conjunction with Education Supervisors. It is a major undertaking, of course, to support tutors and supervisors at grassroots level, because their position and seniority of ten means they are unlikely to have experienced the relevant leadership training themselves. Chapters 4–11 are an example of this support offered as various learning options for doctors at all and each career stage.

Alongside the educational processes, further support for learners and tutors has been developed in the form of e-learning material. The Academy of Medical Royal Colleges, in conjunction with e-Learning for Healthcare (eLfH), have developed 50×20-minute learning units that provide the background and theoretical underpinnings to the MLCF; this also includes various examples of the competences in practice. All this material is available free to all those with a GMC registration.

BPP
LEARNING MEDIA

Further developments

The positive reception given to the MLCF and acceptance of the appropriateness of its content are reflected in two recent developments. First, the NHS Institute for Innovation and Improvement was commissioned to consider whether the MLCF could be adapted for use by other clinical professions. The consultation received a very positive response, with all clinical groups endorsing the framework and wishing to see it incorporated into their own training and development. This incorporation is now underway, enabling all clinicians to have a common basis and language in their development as clinical leaders. Furthermore, the five original domains of the MLCF have now been adopted as the basis of the NHS Leadership Framework. This framework describes the leadership basis for all staff working in the healthcare sector, both public and private. Two further domains have been added to the original five and are directed to the relatively small group of staff in designated, positional leadership roles. It is encouraging, then, to recognise that as doctors acquire the competences of the MLCF described in this chapter, they also acquire the basis of leadership used by all other staff, including managers and executives.

A final development has seen the establishment of a new Faculty of Medical Leadership and Management (FMLM). This is an organisation aimed at bringing together various initiatives in medical leadership and acting as a focus for developments in the areas of education, support networks and research. It is a body endorsed by all Medical Royal Colleges and has a Council drawn from constituent colleges. It spans the profession from undergraduate and postgraduate, through to revalidation and national medical leaders. It also seeks to be a membership organisation – again reflecting the spectrum of the medical profession.

References

British Association of Medical Managers (BAMM) (2007) *A Syllabus for Doctors in Management and Leadership Positions in Healthcare*. Manchester, UK: BAMM.

General Medical Council (GMC) (2006) *Management for Doctors*. Manchester, UK: General Medical Council.

General Medical Council (2009) *Tomorrow's Doctors: Recommendations on undergraduate medical education*. [Online] Manchester, UK: GMC. Available at www.gmc-uk.org/education/undergraduate/tomorrows_doctors_2009. asp [Accessed 17/10/11].

Ham C and Dickinson H. (2007) *Engaging Doctors in Leadership: A review of the literature*. Coventry: NHS Institute for Innovation and Improvement.

Lucia A D and Lepsinger R (1999) *The Art and Science of Competency Models: pinpointing critical success factors in organisations*. San Francisco, CA: Jossey Bass.

McKenna M, Gartland P and Pugno P. Development of physician leadership competencies: perceptions of physician leaders, physician educators and medical students. *The Journal of Health Administration Education* 2004; 21(3) pp. 343–54.

NHS Institute for Innovation and Improvement and Academy of Medical Royal Colleges (2010) *Medical Leadership Competency Framework*. 3rd edition. Coventry: NHS Institute for Innovation and Improvement. p. 6.

The Royal College of Physicians (2005) *Doctors in society: medical professionalism in a changing world*. Report of a Working Party of the Royal College of Physicians of London. London: RCP.

The Royal College of Physicians and Surgeons of Canada (RPCSP) (2005) *The CanMEDS Project Overview*. Ottawa: RCPSP.

Wass V and Van der Vleuten C. (2009) Assessment in Medical Education and Training. In Carter Y and Jackson N (eds.) *Medical Education and Training: from theory to delivery*. Oxford: Oxford University Press. p. 105.

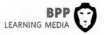

Chapter 3

Management and Leadership

Peter Spurgeon

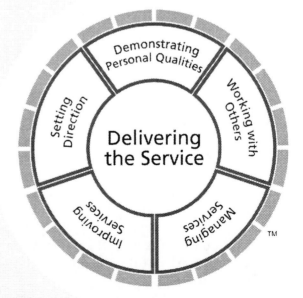

Management and Leadership

 Chapter overview

This chapter provides:

- A discussion of the distinction between management and leadership
- An understanding of the various models and approaches to leadership
- An explanation of the model of Shared Leadership that underpins the Medical Leadership Competency Framework

Introduction

The previous chapters have illustrated the importance attached to medical leadership across many health systems; of particular relevance here is the UK's response, with the development and dissemination of the Medical Leadership Competency Framework (MLCF). However, it may be worth noting that most of the advocates have commented that very little attention has been paid to two particular conceptual views which often provoke debate, if not confusion and misunderstanding. These two issues are:

1. Should management be clearly differentiated from leadership?
2. When we use the term leadership, are we (authors, commentators and readers) all using it to mean exactly the same thing?

A number of well established texts discuss these issues at length; see Hartley and Benington, *Leadership for Healthcare* (2010) or Spurgeon, Clark and Ham, *Medical Leadership: from the dark side to centre stage* (2011). It is not the intention here to discuss these issues in great depth. The overall aim of this book is to support practice in the use and implementation of the MLCF. However, previous experience suggests that questions – often coming from the sceptical end of the profession – may well arise in the context of these two issues and it is therefore helpful to be armed with a few discussion points.

Management or leadership?

There are several issues embedded here. For example, is it possible to draw a clear distinction between the two terms? Does it matter whether or not this is possible? In terms of the latter, there may well be some significant assumptions about the two concepts that make them inherently more or less attractive activities. If the history of the NHS is traced in terms of organisational models, it is possible to see its evolution from an administered service to a managed one and currently, to one where leadership is the main currency. The role of doctors within these different organisational paradigms has changed. At the outset, the function of the administrative role was to support the doctor and both parties saw this as a subsidiary role. The new management movement of the 1980s and 1990s was based on the principle of enhanced accountability, ostensibly to embrace the medical profession within the managed process. But this was mostly unsuccessful and spawned many interprofessional divisions, as each tried to establish its influence and authority. The most recent model has been to seek to invite all staff groups to contribute within a broad concept of leadership. It is worth noting that the latter has, so far, proved more successful in attracting doctors to participate in the running of their organisation. It is probably sensible to conclude, then, that the distinction between management and leadership *can* matter.

The stereotype of managers, or management, probably plays into this perspective with individuals feeling resentful about being managed and perceiving management to be inherently bureaucratic and controlling. In contrast, the *charismatic leader*, articulating a positive vision of the future, is a rather more appealing prospect. Spurgeon and Cragg discuss this distinction and emphasise the implications for training individuals, depending on whether it is a management task or leadership that is being developed. They also emphasise the focus on management or leadership that is partly framed by the context in which the processes operate. To summarise, they suggest that:

> *the basic functions of management – planning, budgeting, organising, controlling resources and problem solving – are vital for the smooth running of any organisation: without them anarchy may result. These managerial activities though are most appropriate when organisations and the society around them are stable and*

BPP
LEARNING MEDIA

> *relatively predictable. The constant and continual change occurring in society and the NHS in particular goes some way to explain why such a premium is placed on leadership. If organisations need to adapt and change to new circumstances then leaders who challenge, motivate and inspire others towards a new vision are critical*

(Spurgeon and Cragg 2007, p. 99)

Perhaps a simplistic summary perspective might be that managers are primarily concerned with making the current system and its procedures operate as efficiently and effectively as possible. Leaders, on the whole, seek to change what currently exists so that the organisation will be better equipped to deal with the future. The latter usually involves a rather longer term perspective and also has a motivational impact upon people who work in the organisation.

The interrelationship of leadership and management

If, as suggested, leadership is regarded as a rather more enticing concept than management (and also essential in times of change), what does this imply for management? Is management seen as a rather more mundane and constrained process, largely overwhelmed by the more powerful and charismatic force of leadership? Or is it actually a component of leadership offering the stable basis on which leadership can develop? The desire for some great definitional distinction between management and leadership may well be a rather pedantic concern; even if the roles are documented as distinct, it makes very little sense in practice. It can lead to the assignment of labels where someone is described as a manager *or* a leader, clearly segregating the roles, often permanently. The following examples may help to make the argument that any distinction between the two quickly becomes blurred in practice.

Organisations will occasionally undertake major overhauls of their policies and practices. This can result in significant changes in work roles, patterns of communication and interdependence between staff groups. The responsibility for change and major implementation programmes will typically fall to a 'manager' and yet the success of the project will often turn on the 'manager's' ability to communicate and convince other staff of the merits of accepting new tasks and goals. This task in itself sounds very like the influencing behaviour that is said to be an essential ingredient of leadership. It may be that some managers find this influencing task very challenging and are not particularly good at it. Such a performance deficit may, for that specific individual, mark a dividing line between their capacity as a manager and their ability to develop and perform as a leader. However, the task itself clearly has aspects of management (ie *planning, structuring, monitoring*) but equally comprises key leadership aspects (ie *communicating, influencing, motivating*).

In a similar but reverse example, a young consultant may seek to set up a new or much improved service. Talking to (ie *influencing*) patients, colleagues and commissioners will be a vital aspect of the work; hence this is considered leadership. But as young doctors who pursue such a goal will quickly recognise, they will be asked to prepare a very detailed business plan to demonstrate the viability of the proposed service development. Few would dispute that the business planning process is a classic management task, therefore, again, this task requires aspects of management and leadership for its success. The point is that **most significant tasks in organisations require aspects of management and leadership**. Individuals will need to move along this dimension as and when task demands change, and some will find the transition difficult. It is not just managers who may find the demands of aspects of leadership challenging – leaders may be able to articulate an inspirational vision but still struggle to put the operational plans in place to enable the organisation to achieve its vision. Perhaps, as Spurgeon and Cragg conclude, it is better to think of management and leadership as processes which interact and support each other, and are both necessary for effective organisations; however, at specific times, one may be emphasised more than the other.

Approaches to leadership

Is it just academic pedantry to question whether the term *leadership* is always used clearly and unambiguously? Or is it actually important in practice to have greater precision and clarity about the term? At a fairly simple level, the definition of leadership may well have implications. Quite frequently trainers and educators will comment that 'everyone can be a leader', or 'leadership is the responsibility of everyone'. Some people hearing this type of statement will, by choice or some sense of self-insight, immediately think 'I am not a leader; I don't want to be.' This quite simple example contains a number of concepts of leadership, which may result in some individuals construing leadership as not for them. It is likely that such individuals will have a rather traditional and stereotypical view of leadership as involving a charismatic, inspirational commanding figure who carries others along by his/her sheer presence. They will then conclude – and probably quite rightly – that they are therefore not a leader. However, this is potentially an inappropriate conclusion, because it is grounded in their particular model of leadership. Therefore it is worth a brief detour into the nature of leadership and the approaches to describing it. Hopefully this will equip the reader with the knowledge and information to understand and perhaps challenge certain statements about leadership.

Leadership models

The study of leadership has existed for many years and has been consistently documented and added to since the 1920s. A particular concern has been with leadership effectiveness, with practitioners seeking answers about the ingredients of success to academics attempting to understand how to demonstrate the impact of leadership. The search to understand leadership has followed a path shaped to a large extent by the nature of society around it at the time. Initially, the focus was on the individual and sought to describe the traits of great successful leaders, reflecting the individualism of entrepreneurship. It then moved to more behavioural approaches, documenting what leaders did, which itself was extended to incorporate details of the context or situation in which leadership occurred. More recently, as society became more complex, democratic and collective, so leadership models attempted to incorporate aspects of complexity and to reflect the impact of education on breaking down conventional social hierarchies. (Please see Northouse (2010), and Hartley and Benington (2010) for good reviews of leadership models.) Many definitions can be found in such texts but the following simple, workable one will be used here: *'when you boil it all down, contemporary leadership seems to be a matter of aligning people towards common goals and empowering them to take the actions needed to reach them'.*

Trait theory

The earliest conceptualisation of leadership focused on trying to identify the traits/characteristics of individuals who, by status, power, achievement, or some form of recognition, were deemed to be leaders. This approach assumed such individuals possessed the vital ingredients that made them leaders. If this could be identified and described it would enable the right people (ie leaders) to be appointed to the appropriate leadership roles. An implicit assumption was that the necessary characteristics would see the same people emerge as leaders across a range of different situations – because they possessed the essential qualities whilst others did not. This theory also regarded these characteristics as innate; people simply had them or did not.

Despite decades of research in pursuit of the key characteristics, the approach has been relatively unsuccessful. Only a few factors (eg superior intelligence, self-confidence, self-starter, extrovert) emerged with any stability across different research contexts. As products of a considerable amount of research, these findings are actually quite meagre and could probably have been specified at the outset. The trait theory, though, lingers partly because people still use their stereotypical model of leadership to judge whether others could be potential leaders, and also because there seems to be some sort of comfort factor in believing in the great leader who will come along and put everything right. This perspective can be seen in the searches conducted by large organisations for a new Chief Executive to restore the fortunes of an ailing company.

Recently, Alimo-Metcalfe developed a more modern and sophisticated model of the trait approach, in her description of engaging leadership. The focus of such work has shifted from the great 'leader' to a more collaborative, participative style, but remains nonetheless a set of character descriptions. The trait theory has produced many lists of qualities, which tend to overlap and universally fail to deal with a number of key questions:

- Are all the characteristics needed in all contexts?
- What combinations are required in particular circumstances?
- How much of any quality does an individual need to possess, ie can great strength in one area compensate for another?

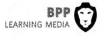

- How in the context of a selection process will classic qualities such as integrity (worthy as it may be) be assessed?

The final deficiencies of the approach stem from the implicit assumption that such characteristics are innate and therefore are largely unable to be acquired. Therefore, if someone does not seem to possess all or certain traits, can they aspire to a leadership role or not? It is also particularly difficult to know what to do with such lists of characteristics. Because of the lack of specificity, how can an individual reconcile positive feelings about some qualities, with negative ones about other? Is it possible to develop the missing characteristics if they are largely regarded as innate? Perhaps the most optimistic and reasonable conclusion is that as it is clear leaders do emerge, then the range of qualities described are probably relevant to some extent; and that leaders will possess a wide variety of combinations of these personal qualities. On this basis, it is possible that everyone can contribute as a leader, but in different ways, with different approaches and by using varying qualities. However, this is unsatisfactory as a research conclusion to an area of study.

Leadership style and context

The relative failure of the personality- or trait-based model saw a shift in focus from who leaders *are* to what they *do*, and the importance of the context in which leadership occurs. Key categories of behaviour which emerged from this strand of research focused on the following:

- Task behaviours: giving a priority to getting the job done
- Relationship behaviours: emphasising the way people work together

The combination and emphasis given to each of these resulted in the concept of leadership *styles*, with debates about whether task and relationship styles could be found in one person alone, or, if necessary, could be fulfilled by separate people. For example, extremely task-focused individuals (often much valued for their level of achievement) will often ride roughshod over the feelings and concerns of others in order to ensure goals are achieved. A more supportive, concerned style was considered to be incompatible with task-achievement and almost impossible to provide simultaneously. However, there is little clear support for these perspectives and indeed a very modern conceptualisation of leadership would now suggest that a supportive, participative style can be the basis of promoting organisational achievement. The aspiration of this research was to link a particular style to outcome, so that the most effective style could be identified; suitable individuals could be offered training and development so that they could work in this way. Once more, however, no such clear relationship could be established.

Instead, the inconsistency of results relating to leadership styles led to a belief that it was the variation in *context* that held the key. This has been described as the *situational* or *contingency* model of leadership. There is a slight difference of emphasis but crucially the idea was that the behaviour of the leader would be more or less appropriate and effective, depending on certain aspects of the context. The degree of competence of the members of the team being led, the rewards available to this follower group and the complexity of the task itself are particularly relevant factors. There has been value in understanding the impact of a range of factors on the success of leader behaviours but it is also fair to say that in trying to establish a degree of certainty about specific leadership-related factors the dynamic inter-play of too many influences has proved rather too complex for clear results.

From individual to collective models

Quite a strong strand of leadership work has formed around the concept of *transactional* versus *transformational* leadership. Aspects of both concepts were presented in earlier parts of this chapter, both in the discussion of management and leadership and of task- or relationship-based leadership styles. *Transactional leadership* is seen as part of a series of exchanges or transactions between a leader and followers, normally based in a hierarchical organisational structure. In contrast, *transformational leadership* does not depend on hierarchy but is a product of followers' desire and willingness to be led by a particular individual. Transformational leadership is based on a personal connection affording influence. As later versions of the transactional/transformational model began to describe, the two are not unlike the managerial (*transactional*)/leadership (*transformational*) dimension described earlier; Bass has described them as being on a continuum. Transformational leadership is generally regarded as the style essential to changing and improving organisations; it has also been associated with greater staff satisfaction, motivation and performance. However, the model still represents an underlying conceptualisation of leadership as based around the individual. A recent model has sought to take a more collective approach to leadership. It is referred to as *shared* or *distributed leadership* and is probably the most persuasive of modern strands.

Shared or distributed leadership

The leadership literature is increasingly recognising that the leader-centric model, where all the focus is on one person, is quite limited. The increasingly complex set of tasks facing organisations has seen a growing reliance on teams; here, leadership tasks are shared across teams, organisational boundaries and networks. Each team member's individual experience, knowledge and capacity is valued and used to distribute or share the job of leadership through the team, in response to each context or challenge being faced. Implicit in this is a realisation that it is unrealistic for one individual to have all the necessary skills. The approach is also inherently more democratic ie it recognises that in a society with higher levels of education, more individuals will be capable of a leadership contribution.

The burgeoning interest in shared leadership chimes well with flatter, less hierarchical organisations which need to respond rapidly and flexibly to continuing change. It gives rise to the advocated position that everyone can make a contribution as a leader at their appropriate level in the organisation. Furthermore, it makes the vital point that is crucial to this entire text: it makes more sense to talk of *leadership* rather than of a *leader*. Leadership consists of a range of behaviours described in the MLCF. These behaviours can be acquired and used at any level in the organisation, and therefore all can contribute leadership (as opposed to leaders) within the relevant part of their organisation.

The MLCF is built upon this model of shared leadership, therefore enabling medical students, postgraduate and experienced doctors to contribute leadership components as the task and context

BPP
LEARNING MEDIA

demands, and as their level in the organisation allows. The next stage is the practical steps all members of the profession can take to acquire and develop skills through implementation of the MLCF, as detailed in Chapters 4–11.

References

Alimo-Metcalfe B and Alban-Metcalfe T. The development of a new transformational leadership questionnaire. *Journal of Occupational and Organisational Psychology.* 2001; 74, pp. 1–27.

Bass B (1998) *Transformational Leadership.* Mahwah, NJ: Lawrence Erlbaum Associates.

Hartley J and Benington J (2010) *Leadership for Healthcare.* Bristol, UK: The Policy Press.

Northouse PG (2010) *Leadership: Theory and Practice.* 5th edition. Thousand Oaks, CA: Sage.

Sherman S. How tomorrow's best leaders are learning their stuff. *Fortune* 1995; 27: 91–92.

Spurgeon P and Cragg R (2007) Is it management or leadership? In Chambers R, Mohanna K, Spurgeon P and Wall D (eds.) *How to Succeed as a Leader.* Oxford: Radcliffe Publishing. p. 99.

Spurgeon P, Clark J and Ham C (2011) *Medical Leadership: From the Dark Side to Centre Stage.* Oxford: Radcliffe Press.

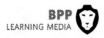

Chapter 4

Leadership Learning on the Wards

Bob Klaber

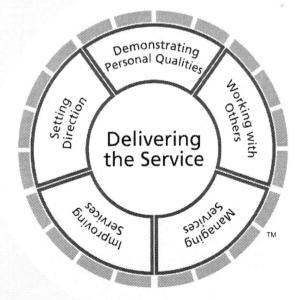

Chapter 4

Leadership Learning on the Wards

 Chapter overview

This chapter examines the opportunities for leadership learning on the wards, and explores a number of key concepts including:

- The culture of feedback on the wards
- Improving continuity of care for patients
- How flattened hierarchies can lead to safer care
- The value of incorporating the nursing perspective
- Involvement of junior doctors as agents of change
- Integrated care pathways

 This chapter also looks at practical tools and techniques which can be used to support learning. These include:

- Techniques for teaching and learning where time is limited
- Upside-down ward rounds to develop decision-making skills
- After Action Reviews (AARs) to look back at team performance
- Checklists to improve patient care

Introduction

A huge amount of medical student and trainee doctor time is spent learning different aspects of clinical medicine on the hospital wards. While maximising the opportunities to develop history-taking, examination, clinical decision-making and procedural skills are paramount, the wards also provide a rich environment for medical students and doctors of all levels to acquire and develop their leadership skills and experiences. The ward environment is the very essence of hospital-based medicine, with different teams working together to provide care and support for patients and their families. This includes the nursing team based on the ward; different medical and surgical teams; multiprofessional teams supporting chronic, complex or specialist care; and other task-based teams such as the pain team, the discharge planning team or the community nursing team. The complexity is huge – this means that as well as being a rich environment in which to learn, it is also an area where there is a high risk of adverse events and errors.

BPP
LEARNING MEDIA

Many medical students and junior doctors have very variable memories of their different ward round experiences. The historical ward round of over twenty participants, each following the regal-like consultant as they stride past their patients, has never been a convincing method for maximising learning nor ensuring high quality care for patients. Yet, to different extents, many of these practices exist on our hospital wards today. Teaching and learning opportunities are frequently missed, and different teams do not always work cohesively together. There are occasions where communication with patients is not as good as it could be, and more often than not the documentation of the *thinking* behind decisions is poor.

This chapter uses the key domains of the MLCF as a broad structure to explore different leadership learning opportunities that can occur on the ward. These examples are by no means exhaustive, but will hopefully provide a stimulus for medical students, junior doctors, or those in a training role, to look at their ward working environment to seek out opportunities for learning and improvement.

Demonstrating Personal Qualities on the wards

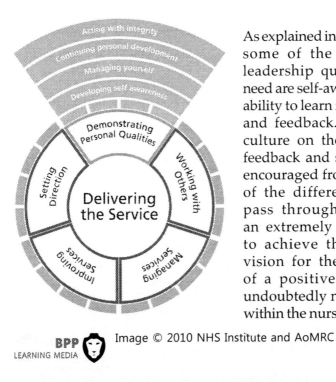

As explained in earlier chapters, some of the key personal leadership qualities doctors need are self-awareness and the ability to learn from experience and feedback. Developing a culture on the ward, where feedback and suggestions are encouraged from all members of the different teams that pass through the ward, is an extremely powerful way to achieve this. While the vision for the development of a positive ward culture undoubtedly needs to be held within the nursing and medical

Image © 2010 NHS Institute and AoMRC

leads, there are a number of ways in which junior members of the team can influence the culture. If successful, this can lead to a richer learning environment, greater staff satisfaction and productivity, and ultimately safer and higher quality patient care.

Exercise 4.1   Scenario

Dr H is a Specialty Training (Year 2) doctor who has been working in the Care of the Elderly department for the last two months. He noticed that there is a great sense of frustration amongst the four consultants within the department because, with all the junior doctors working shifts, there is very little continuity of care for the chronically ill, complex patients who typically spend several weeks on the ward. As a result, there is a significant amount of standing around on ward rounds, with little contribution to any discussion or decision-making from the junior members of the team. In addition, discharge summaries are often not done, or are of poor quality, and there is a general acceptance within the medical team that this is inevitable because of the disjointed nature of the rota.

- How could Dr H go about tacking these different issues?
- Who would Dr H need to involve in any discussions and planning?
- How might Dr H know if he had been successful?

Summary of issues

In this example, Dr H has identified a number of issues which inhibit a positive learning culture on his ward, and are likely to actively compromise the delivery of safe patient care. The reduction in doctors' working hours from the working practices of the 20th century has reduced the risks associated with overtired junior doctors performing tasks beyond their level of competence. However, loss of continuity of patient knowledge is a significant issue for patient care. Additionally, this has also contributed to the disengagement of some junior doctors with no personal feeling of 'ownership' of the ward, where previously a junior doctor may have known every last detail of each of the patients on it.

Improving continuity

In this scenario, these issues could be tackled in several ways. With larger numbers of junior doctors working fewer hours, it is unrealistic to expect one junior member of the team to solely provide the continuity. However, it may be possible to pair up members of the team to take on 'continuity responsibilities' for particular patients. This may work out best as a junior doctor/ nurse pairing, as a pairing of two junior doctors of different levels, or as any other combination from within the multiprofessional team. This is also an excellent opportunity to bring medical and nursing students into this type of learning activity. This 'named pair' could be asked to take the lead on a wide range of tasks which may include supporting discharge planning, linking in with community services and primary care, and working to support the emotional and psychological wellbeing of the patient and their family. Whether it is within the context of a morning ward round, or within a multiprofessional clinical meeting, each 'named pair' could present their case(s) to other members of the team. This provides an excellent opportunity for multiprofessional input into patient care, alongside constructive feedback for the presenting pair and wider learning for the whole team. When open feedback becomes such a regular occurrence that it is the norm, students and trainees feel 'safe' in their working environment, and can contribute more fully to maintaining a culture of learning and self-development. Names are another key aspect in supporting colleagues to feel valued; ensuring that, at each patient's bedside, every single member of the team is introduced by name to the patient and their family is a simple and quick intervention. This can have an extremely positive effect on how a team works, and crucially on how a patient and their family feel they can communicate with the medical team.

Teaching and learning where time is limited

While these sort of initiatives are hard to argue against, the pressure of time is a much cited barrier to learning, and can mean that there is sometimes an acceptance from both teacher (trainer) and learner (trainee or student) that there is too much going on in a ward round to be able to teach. There are a number of teaching tools that help challenge this notion; perhaps the best known of these is the One-Minute Preceptor model (Furney *et al.*, 2001; Irby and Wilkerson,

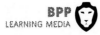

2008). Originally introduced as the 'Five-Step "Microskills" Model of Clinical Teaching' (Neher *et al.*, 1992), the One-Minute Preceptor was developed to illustrate that, even within 60 seconds, a learner, provided they were prepared to commit to some thinking, could be facilitated through the following six steps in order to elucidate an aspect of learning. As illustrated in the flowchart below, the model asks the learner to commit to an answer before critically evaluating their own response. It is then the teacher's responsibility to provide constructive feedback to the learner, and to tease out a general principle that may be of use on another occasion.

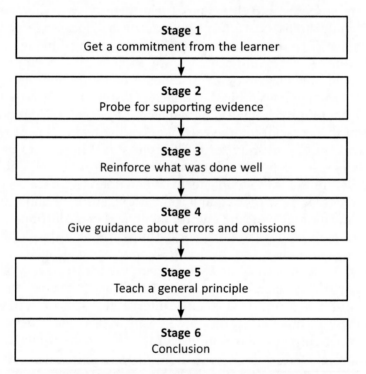

Figure 4.1 The One-Minute Preceptor Model

This method, and others like it, can be used to support both clinical and other non-clinical domains of learning. If embedded within the culture of ward activities such as rounds, multidisciplinary meetings and handover, tools and techniques like these can influence a positive learning culture and support the development of key personal qualities in all members of the team.

Working with Others on the wards

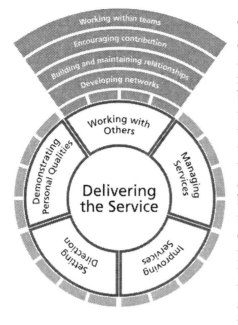

The development of a culture of learning and feedback within a ward setting not only has an impact on personal qualities, but is also crucial to successful teamwork. As described earlier, there is great complexity from the different teams that work within the ward environment, and this is often exacerbated by the historical hierarchies that effectively dictate who can talk to who. The big problem with this setup is that it creates an environment where junior members of teams are discouraged to think for themselves and are less likely to highlight any practices they have noted as unsafe, inefficient or sub-optimal.

One of the key elements of the *Working with Others* MLCF domain is to encourage the contribution of others. It describes listening, supporting others, gaining trust and showing understanding; therefore creating an environment where others have the opportunity to contribute.

Exercise 4.2   **Scenario**

Dr Y is a Consultant Paediatrician who, during his attending week, leads a daily ward round to review the patients who have been admitted under his care. Most patients are only admitted for less than 24–48 hours before being ambulated, thought there are a few chronic, complex patients who will be inpatients for the whole week and beyond. While the ward round runs reasonably smoothly, Dr Y reflects on three important issues he feels could be improved:

> **Exercise 4.2** *(Continued)* **Scenario**
>
> 1. The junior doctors on the ward round always look to him to make any decisions, and will only rarely contribute to the thinking around decision-making.
> 2. Although he tries to encourage contribution from more junior members of the team, he reflects that it is unlikely any of them would point out a mistake that he might make.
> 3. The nursing staff are so overstretched that it is very unusual for them to be on the ward round, and he is concerned about the impact this has on teamwork and communication.
>
> - How could Dr Y go about tackling these three issues?
> - How might Dr Y know if he had been successful?

Summary of issues

The exercise above illustrates some of the problems that occur in varying degrees in wards across different specialties and hospitals. The historical hierarchies of hospital medicine established themselves at a time where all of the input into a patient's care came solely through the patient's named consultant. The different doctors under the consultant were there to learn and carry out the actions from these decisions. The opinion of the patient carried much less weight than it does today and there was little emphasis on multiprofessional working. While there is clearly some benefit to the clarity of decision-making that this historical model ensured, it is somewhat surprising that, in some departments, many elements of this way of working remain entirely unchanged.

Dr Y's reflections in the exercise above illustrate a scenario where a senior doctor recognises the opportunity to improve teamwork within the ward. Although any improvements will need the approval of senior doctors and ward managers, many of the ideas discussed and others like them could be initiated and evaluated by junior team members.

Developing decision-making skills

In many specialties there has been a significant move towards consultant-delivered care to improve both health outcomes and the experience of patients. However, this is only a sustainable

BPP
LEARNING MEDIA

approach within the NHS if senior doctors continue to support and develop their junior colleagues in their learning. One of the most important aspects of learning is to be put in a position where you can weigh up the evidence available from the history, examination and investigations to formulate a differential diagnosis and make a decision about a management plan. This is the fulcrum of clinical medicine, yet so often junior doctors and medical students are not asked to do the thinking and make the decisions. Clearly, within the context of a consultant-led service, there is a need to use checks and 'safety nets' where a consultant reviews these decisions prior to their implementation. However, too often the junior doctors and medical students on the wards are excluded from participating in meaningful thinking and decision-making before a plan is made.

One of the most straightforward ways to overcome this issue is to establish an 'upside-down ward round'. This means turning the usual roles of the ward round on their head. In Dr Y's paediatric example he, as the consultant, can write the notes while watching how the rest of the team perform in their roles. The Registrar can review observation records and drug charts, the Senior House Officer can examine the patient, and the Foundation Year doctor can introduce the team to the family and go through the relevant aspects of the history. Depending upon the complexity of the case one of the junior team members can formulate a management plan and explain this to the family. The consultant can then back up this management plan or amend it as necessary.

Normal ward round		Task		Upside-down ward round
Foundation year doctor	⇐	Write in notes (and watch rest of team)	⇒	Consultant
SHO	⇐	Review obs records and drug charts	⇒	SpR
SpR/Consultant	⇐	Examine the patient	⇒	SHO
Consultant	⇐	Introduce team and explore history	⇒	Foundation Year doctor
Consultant	⇐	Formulate management plan and explain to patient/family	⇒	Junior member of team

Figure 4.2 The 'upside-down ward round'

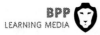

This provides opportunities for the consultant to role-model the quality of documentation in patient notes that is expected, to perform workplace-based assessments and to give constructive feedback to the different team members. It may be that this works best for certain patients, or ward rounds on certain days of the week, but as a simple technique it provides an important way of actively involving all members of the team in decision-making.

Flattening hierarchies

Initiatives such as the 'upside-down ward round' have an important secondary effect of flattening the historical hierarchy described above. While a doctor who has been recently appointed as a consultant may superficially feel that, after years of being on the receiving end of orders coming down the hierarchy, it is now their turn to do the shouting, this approach is highly illogical. A flatter hierarchy of teamworking, where any member of the team, be they a junior doctor or student nurse, can highlight a problem, flag an impending error or feedback a patient's concerns is likely to lead to the delivery of much safer and higher quality care. This conversation may take the form of an informal discussion between patients on the ward round, or in a more structured framework such as an After Action Review (discussed in more detail in the 'Managing Services' section).

The nursing perspective

In the exercise above Dr Y's final reflection was around the difficulty the nursing team had in finding the time to join the ward round. To understand this issue, it is essential to talk to the ward manager and both the junior and senior nurses to establish the problems. It may be that the ward rounds are perceived as a 'doctor-only' arena, or that they are an inefficient use of nursing time. Perhaps the nurses feel they learn very little from the experience, or that it is frustrating waiting around for the medical team to get to each of the different patients an individual nurse is looking after. A clearer understanding of the nursing perspective may produce straightforward solutions. Doctors traditionally approach ward rounds from Bed 1 to Bed 24, but a strategy where the most unwell patients are seen first, followed by all of the patients who are likely to be discharged, may be more efficient. An individual nurse may be looking after three or four patients spread across different areas of the ward. Finding any of the nurses who are free at the beginning of the ward round and seeing their three or four patients first, before finding a second nurse and then seeing their three or four patients, etc, might be a way towards resolving this problem.

Managing Services on the wards

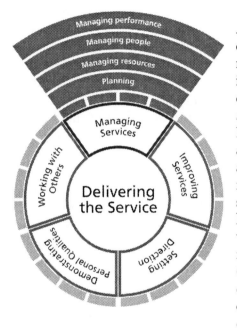

Another important leadership competency focuses on managing people, and this is one of the four elements detailed within the *Managing Services* domain of the MLCF. Doctors show leadership in this area by providing guidance and direction for others, reviewing performance and supporting others to provide high quality patient care. The well established processes for educational supervision (Klaber *et al.*, 2010) for trainee doctors in the UK are an example of formal processes designed to support this area.

As well as using educational supervision to guide their own continuing personal development and learning needs throughout their training, junior doctors also need to take steps to develop their own supervisory skills. After postgraduate training the majority of doctors will have a supervisory role over junior colleagues, which is a significant responsibility that requires time and specific skills.

After Action Reviews (AARs)

There are other approaches to looking back at team activities which move on from reviewing performance to developing a learning critique. The After Action Review (AAR) takes a retrospective team-based view on an episode, or series of events, to support team members in developing their roles and responsibilities in working together to deliver good patient care. AARs were first used by the US Army in the 1970s and then spread to industry and business in the 1990s. They aim to encourage feedback up and down hierarchy levels by creating 'safe' times, when criticisms and suggestions can be aired by everyone involved in a project or episode (Collison and Parcell, 2001). Many businesses have credited them as being a helpful technique in transforming a top-down authoritative culture into a two-way collaborative culture, even where management structures remain unchanged. They are now also being used by a number of healthcare organisations across the world, and are the sort of tool that can offer significant support to leadership learning within the context of a ward (Connecting for Health, 2010). Some healthcare organisations have taken a systematic approach to training large numbers of their workforce in this technique so that AARs can be implemented at different levels throughout the organisation. While there are formal mechanisms for setting up and running an AAR, perhaps the most useful aspect of this technique is the informal approach, which can easily be applied to almost any aspect of teamworking on a ward. Quite simply, each member of the team who was involved in a particular event (eg a discussion with a patient, a resuscitation, a handover) answers four questions:

1. What was supposed to happen?
2. What actually happened?
3. Why were there differences?
4. What did we learn?

These questions can be answered on an individual level as a personal reflection, or as a group activity where everyone's thoughts are brought together by one member of the team who acts as facilitator. This is a role that can be taken on by any member of the team – their responsibility is in guiding the team to get the most possible learning from the review.

Improving Services on the wards

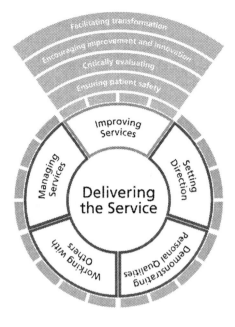

One feature of successful healthcare organisations is their ability to get the most out of junior doctors in terms of contributing to service improvements. The frequent rotations (usually between 3-monthly and 12-monthly) of trainees in and out of a particular hospital department can dilute any sense of organisational belonging doctors in training may have, but there are advantages of fresh perspectives and experience from other organisations that can be used to great effect.

However, too often trainees are never asked about their previous experiences, what worked well in their previous NHS Trust or how they think improvements to patient care could be made. If they are given the appropriate space and support, the wards are an excellent clinical area where junior doctors and medical students can think about, plan and implement improvements. A simple example of an improvement project that could be adopted in a ward setting is illustrated in Exercise 4.3.

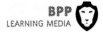

Exercise 4.3   **Scenario**

Dr A is a Specialty Trainee doctor in Paediatrics, who works with Dr Y from Exercise 4.2. She has recently been involved in an episode where her prescription for antibiotics was mis-read by one of the nursing team, and the wrong dose was administered to a patient. She is very upset by this episode and wants to learn all she can from this mistake. On talking to the lead pharmacist she learns that these prescribing errors are extremely common. She realises that while there are many safety checks and initiatives to reduce the chance of dispensing errors (by pharmacists) and administration errors (by nurses) of medicines, the majority of doctors have a very laidback attitude to prescribing. Doctors are often asked to amend drug charts while dealing with other tasks on a ward round, and for many, the writing of a new drug chart is considered to be a boring 'copying' task. Dr A resolves to try to improve this situation by developing a strategy to re-focus the minds of her and her colleagues on the importance of safe prescribing.

- What key issues does Dr A need to address?
- What sort of interventions might help her to do this?
- How might she know if her intervention has made any difference?

Summary of issues

This exercise highlights an important patient safety issue, and one common to all specialties. Extensive research demonstrates the widespread patient harm associated with imperfect prescribing. There are a number of approaches Dr A might take to make these improvements to safe prescribing. One of the simplest methods is the use of the humble checklist.

Checklists

If your initial reaction to reading the word 'checklist' is to think that this is far too basic an idea for something as complex as healthcare, it is worth reading Atul Gawande's highly thought-provoking book, *The Checklist Manifesto* (2009). Gawande is a general and endocrine surgeon at the Brigham and Women's Hospital in Boston, US, who has led the World Health Organization's 'Safe Surgery Saves Lives

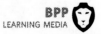

Challenge'. He argues that checklists could bring about striking improvements throughout medicine, and challenges those who think checklists are beneath them:

> *The fear people have about the idea of adherence to protocol is rigidity. They imagine mindless automatons, heads down in a checklist, incapable of looking out ... and coping with the real world in front of them. But what you find, when a checklist is well made, is exactly the opposite. The checklist gets the dumb stuff out of the way, the routines your brain shouldn't have to occupy itself with .... and lets it rise above to focus on the hard stuff.*

(Gawande, 2009)

Gawande describes how applying this idea to surgery has produced a 90-second checklist that, at virtually no cost, has reduced deaths and complications by more than 33% in eight hospitals around the world. The issues that Dr A has unpicked around prescribing could also be addressed by a checklist that junior doctors could use on the daily ward round. Using this technique has made significant improvements on an Acute Medical Unit (Caldwell, 2010). Figure 4.3 shows one example of a checklist is currently used on a paediatric ward. The idea is that this checklist is 'owned' by the junior medical staff who, during every daily ward round, review the drug chart of every patient on the ward against the checklist. Any omissions or errors are corrected at the time, and the 'checker', who could also be a medical student, feeds back common themes to the medical team. Gawande is clear that in order to be successful checklists should be focused on where the evidence shows error to occur, and their content should be frequently revisited and redesigned.

Ward X – Daily inpatient prescribing checklist

Instructions: This checklist should be completed by one of the medical team during the daily ward round. 'Tick' if the chart is completely correct, and 'cross' if it is imperfect, unclear or missing information.

		Bedspace:	1	2	3	4	5	6	7	8
		Bedspace occupied (Y or N)?								
		Patient initials								
Front page	Patient name on front page									
	Date of birth on front page									
	Hospital number on front page									
	Name of ward on front page									
	Name of consultant on front page									
	Admission weight on front page									
	Completed allergy box on front page (including the type of any reaction)									
Medicines	All drugs prescribed legibly									
	All doses clear with unambiguous units									
	All drug frequencies clearly prescribed									
	All drug timings clear and unambiguous									
	All drug routes clearly detailed									
	All prescriptions signed for with name of doctor printed in CAPITAL letters									
Abx	Indication for any antibiotics detailed									
	Actual start date for antibiotics detailed									
	Planned duration for antibiotics detailed									
Fluids	All fluid prescriptions clear with which fluid, volume of bag, additives, rate & signature									
	Is the drug chart 100% correct?									

Date: Completed by:

% of charts

Learning points (including recurrent issues & themes):

Figure 4.3 Prescribing checklist for use on ward rounds

If they are well planned, and have the approval of senior doctors and ward staff, then a simple checklist has great potential to make significant improvements to patient care.

Setting Direction on the wards

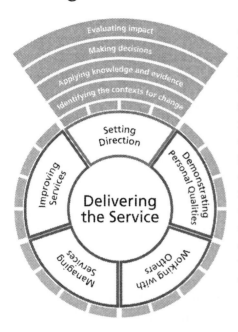

This is the fifth domain of the MLCF, and at first glance it may seem the most difficult area for enthusiastic medical students, or junior doctors early in their careers, to influence change. This area of leadership focuses on identifying the contexts for change; applying relevant knowledge and evidence; participating in and contributing to organisational decision-making processes; and then evaluating the impact of changes made.

No-one would expect a junior member of a clinical team to make key strategic decisions for the organisation they work for. However, the experiences that junior doctors gain of working on the frontline within different organisations, of close patient contact, of different teams and different ways of working give them a powerful perspective on the context for change. The key is for healthcare organisations, who benefit from the influx of new junior doctors every three, six or twelve months, to find mechanisms and opportunities to learn from the unique perspectives trainees bring.

Integrated care pathways

The development and evaluation of integrated care pathways is one example of an area of change that junior doctors should be immersed in throughout their training. Integrated care pathways

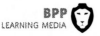

were introduced in the early 1990s in the UK and the US, and have since grown to become a key component of many health systems, including the NHS. They are perhaps best described as structured, multidisciplinary care plans designed to support the implementation of clinical guidelines and protocols (Campbell *et al.*, 1998; Hill, 1998).

> *Integrated Care Pathways define the expected course of events in the care of a patient with a particular condition, within a set time-scale. A pathway is divided into time intervals during which specific goals and expected progress are defined, together with appropriate investigations and treatment. A pathway reflects the activities of a multidisciplinary team and can incorporate established guidelines and evidence-based medicine.*

(Kitchiner *et al.*, 1996)

As healthcare looks to work in a heavily integrated way across the traditional primary-secondary care interface, the idea of integrated care pathways takes on a further dimension. Studies are beginning to emerge that demonstrate, for specific conditions, that a general practice-led model of integrated care can significantly reduce outpatient attendance and improve patient experience while maintaining the quality of care (Julian *et al.*, 2007). Policy changes in the UK, which give the responsibility for commissioning the majority of healthcare to General Practitioners (GPs), are likely to further encourage the development of these initiatives.

Contributing their experiences and thinking to the development of these pathways is likely to give junior doctors valuable experience in understanding the role of national guidelines (eg from the National Institute for Health and Clinical Excellence [NICE]) and frameworks (eg National Service Framework [NSF]). Involvement in patient pathway work will also expose them to patient experience data and other activity data from which a 'case for change' can be made. They will also have the opportunity to meet and talk to the teams responsible for the commissioning of services, and so will garner a greater understanding of how different services are established and paid for.

Summary

With their complexity and variety of activity, hospital wards provide a hugely rich environment for all members of the medical team, from medical students to consultants, to develop their leadership skills and experiences. We have considered a number of important concepts around flattening hierarchies, creating a 'safe' learning culture and using junior doctors as 'agents for change'. These ideas will run through all of the remaining chapters of the book. We have also explained the role of several different tools and techniques including the One-Minute Preceptor, After Action Reviews, checklists and integrated care pathways. The challenge for us all is to now go out and start making things happen.

 Three things to try

1. Break with old habits and turn one of your ward rounds 'upside-down' so different people take on different roles. Think about how you might better involve nursing colleagues.
2. When you next teach, think about how you can create a learning culture where learners feel comfortable to commit to answers without fear of being wrong.
3. Design and implement a checklist to improve patient safety or efficiency in one of your clinical areas.

References

Caldwell G. Real Time 'Check and Correct' of Drug Charts on Ward Rounds. *Pharmacy Management* 2010; 26(4): 3–9.

Campbell H *et al.* Integrated care pathways. *BMJ (Clinical Research Ed.)* 1998; 316(7125): 133–137.

Collison C and Parcell G (2001) Chapter 10: Networking and communities of practice. In *Learning to fly: practical lessons from one of the world's leading knowledge companies.* Oxford: Capstone.

Connecting for Health (2010) After Action Review [Online] Available at www.connecting for health. nhs.uk/ systems and services/ icd/ knowledge/ kmtools/ cards/ aar.pdf [Accessed 30/10/11].

Furney SL *et al.* Teaching the one-minute preceptor. A randomized controlled trial. *Journal of General Internal Medicine* 2001; 16(9): 620–624.

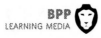

Gawande A (2009) *The Checklist Manifesto: How to Get Things Right*. New York, US: Henry Holt and Co.

Hill M. The development of care management systems to achieve clinical integration. *Advanced Practice Nursing Quarterly* 1998; 4(1): 33–39.

Irby DM and Wilkerson L. Teaching when time is limited. *BMJ* 2008; 336(7640): 384–387.

Julian S *et al.* An integrated care pathway for menorrhagia across the primary-secondary interface: patients' experience, clinical outcomes, and service utilisation. *Quality & Safety in Health Care* 2007; 16(2): 110–115.

Kitchiner D, Davidson C and Bundred P. Integrated care pathways: effective tools for continuous evaluation of clinical practice. *Journal of Evaluation in Clinical Practice* 1996; 2(1): 65–69.

Klaber RE, Mellon AF and Melville CA. Educational supervision. *Archives of Disease in Childhood – Education & Practice Edition* 2010; 95: 124–130.

Neher JO *et al.* A five-step "microskills" model of clinical teaching. *The Journal of the American Board of Family Practice/American Board of Family Practice* 1992; 5(4): 419–424.

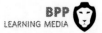

Chapter 5

Leadership Learning in Clinic

Bob Klaber

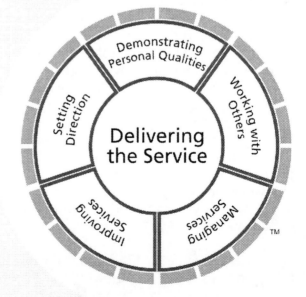

Chapter 5

Leadership Learning in Clinic

 ### *Chapter overview*

This chapter examines the opportunities for leadership learning in clinic, and explores a number of key concepts including:

- The different administrative, managerial and clinic roles
- Improving efficiency through reducing 'Did Not Attend' (DNA) rates regarding appointments
- Using patient feedback to drive forward improvements to services
- Developing alternatives to the traditional out-patient model

 This chapter also looks at practical tools and techniques which can be used to support learning. These include:

- The use of Multi-Source Feedback (MSF)
- Shadowing patients on their 'journey' through outpatients
- Pairing up clinicians and managers in a peer-learning scheme

---

Introduction

A huge amount of clinical care for patients of all ages, and with almost all conditions, is delivered in an outpatient or clinic setting. Although the delivery of care can be planned in a way that is not possible on a ward or within A&E, with every department often simultaneously running any number of different clinic lists, it is an extremely complex system. It is estimated that between May 2009 and April 2010 there were over 84 million outpatient appointments made in NHS hospitals in England; of these, 6.7 million (7.9%) were not attended by the patient (The NHS Information Centre, 2010).

With these huge numbers, and the varied patient needs of each consultation, the complexity is stark. However, the high levels of activity in outpatients also provide a great opportunity – any innovation or improvement, no matter how small, can be multiplied out to have a wide impact that improves care for a large number of patients.

One recent change to how doctors run outpatient clinics has followed the implementation of the European Working Time

Directive, which reduced the working week of junior doctors to an average of less than 48 hours per week (Department of Health, 2004). Departments have responded to this reduction in working hours by re-configuring junior doctor rotas to ensure there is sufficient out-of-hours emergency cover for their services. The knock-on effect is that most medical trainees spend considerably less time working and learning in outpatient settings than they did previously. From a patient's perspective this a good thing (that most outpatient care is delivered by consultants), but there is a danger that with so little exposure to clinics during training, the consultants of tomorrow will be much less experienced at delivering care in this setting. This issue needs to be tackled by innovative rotas, the establishment of training clinics where junior doctors are supervised running outpatient sessions, and a level of self-direction from medical trainees to grab every opportunity they can to gain clinic experience. The parallels with the fewer hours of operating time available to surgical trainees are strong – this issue is discussed in Chapter 8.

In this chapter, we will again use the five domains of the MLCF as a broad structure to explore different leadership learning opportunities that can occur in clinic. Many of the ideas are also applicable to other clinical areas. We hope this chapter will inspire medical students, junior doctors and those in a training role to think about finding opportunities for learning and improvement within outpatients or other clinic settings.

Demonstrating Personal Qualities in clinic

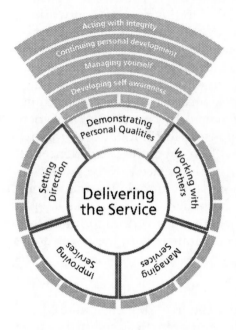

Perhaps the most important aspect of personal leadership development for any doctor is the ability to identify their own strengths and limitations; to recognise the impact of their behaviour on others; and to understand how pressure and stress affect their behaviour. There are many different ways to go about achieving this self-awareness, though the majority are underpinned by the concept of *feedback*. In Chapter 4 we focused on some of the advantages of having a flattened team hierarchy.

Feedback is another area which can become much more meaningful and useful to team members where there is a genuine feeling of openness to talk to each other. With the skills and experience doctors have of difficult conversations with patients and their families, it would seem that a culture of feedback amongst doctors and other health professionals should be easy to achieve. However, the reality is often very different. The well established culture where people give criticisms and comments predominantly behind people's backs has proved difficult to overcome, despite many different initiatives to establish a reflective, learning culture within the healthcare system.

Multi-source feedback (MSF)

One of the most significant moves to engender a reflective, learning culture has come through the introduction of *multi-source feedback* or *360-degree feedback*. One of the earliest times that written surveys were used to gather information about employees occurred in the 1950s at the Esso Research and Engineering Company (Bracken *et al.*, 1997). In the 1990s more businesses began to support the development of their employees with processes of 360-degree

Image © 2010 NHS Institute and AoMRC

feedback, although the processes involved were often very cumbersome. It was not until the early part of the 21st century when, with the rapid development of the internet, the possibility of using web-based electronic surveys became a reality. Since then most medical training programs have instituted annual multi-source feedback to help inform on the progress of an individual through training. Many employers also use them as part of the annual appraisal process for senior clinicians. Some rely on scoring systems, whilst others are focused on a developmental agenda and attempt to collate more qualitative feedback.

Feedback from patients

As well as asking for the comments of other doctors and medical staff, a number of these feedback tools also ask for patient input (Campbell *et al.*, 2010; Lelliott *et al.*, 2008). Outpatient settings are perhaps the ideal place to ask patients about how they think their doctor has performed over a period of time, as surveys can be administered in the time before, or immediately after, a patient is being seen by the doctor. Much of the work to date, which links patient feedback into multi-source feedback tools, has involved supporting the process of consultant appraisal, relicensing and revalidation. As a result the focus of the feedback concentrates on the quantitative assessment of performance rather than on informing learning and development. While it is understandable that the regulatory authorities have headed in this direction, this approach misses a key opportunity: namely that all doctors should be looking to *learn* from their patients' experiences, not just be 'scored' by them. If well presented, feedback can be used to influence individual behaviours as well as leading to improvements in services, a concept discussed in the 'Improving Services' section later in this chapter.

Developing a feedback culture

Junior members of the team can contribute hugely to the establishment of a positive feedback culture. The most effective way of achieving this is for trainees to role-model between themselves the openness, trust and prioritisation of learning that are needed to achieve this feedback culture. Each individual member of the team needs to think about the different opportunities they have to give their colleagues constructive feedback. In most departments

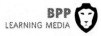

there will be many opportunities every single day – historically, simple observational audits show that these have almost all been missed. Trainees also need to be comfortable with receiving personal feedback themselves, and to develop strategies to implement any of the suggested changes.

Working with Others in clinic

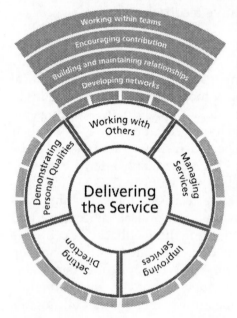

The outpatient setting is an excellent arena to help medical students, and doctors in training, to understand how cohesive teams of clinical and non-clinical staff, working in many different roles, are required to run a clinical service. As a starting point consider the questions in Exercise 5.1.

Exercise 5.1   **Scenario**

Dr R is a Foundation Year doctor who is working in a rheumatology post. Her educational supervisor is keen for her to start developing basic outpatient experience and gain an understanding of the role of different teams in the hospital. She asks Dr R to think about the 'patient journey' that one of her patients takes from the point where her GP refers them to be seen in the hospital.

- What are the different steps that may occur on this 'patient journey'?
- Who are the different people typically involved in these steps?

     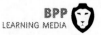

Summary of issues

At first glance the answers to these questions appear to be simple – someone to send out the appointment; a receptionist to welcome the patients and co-ordinate the clinic; and a doctor to see the patient should cover most eventualities.

However, as you may have recognised in your own answers to the questions above, there are many other aspects to an outpatient based clinical service.

Administrative and managerial roles in outpatients

Most clinical services have a team of administrative and clerical staff who take on the role of making and managing appointments, co-ordinating the pulling of notes from medical records, recording clinic activity, and typing and sending out clinic letters. A hospital manager is responsible for this work, and will also co-ordinate the processing and analysis of activity data. Most outpatient services in the NHS are run on a 'payment by results' basis. Within this framework, different clinics have a per-patient payment which they receive for seeing each new patient and a different rate for a follow-up appointment. If the activity is not correctly recorded and processed then the healthcare provider running the clinics will not receive all of the income they are due.

Clinical roles in outpatients

In addition to non-clinical staff there are many different clinical roles that support outpatient work. Outpatient nursing work may involve general nursing skills around measuring observations and weighing patients or very specialist input to support a particular type of clinic. Many clinics are now multidisciplinary and there may be professionals such as psychologists, dieticians, nurse specialists or speech and language therapists working with the doctor. Other staff, such as a play specialist in a children outpatients service, may be there to help support the 'patient experience'. Some clinics are also looking for innovative ways to communicate more effectively with patients and other professionals; consequently there may be staff with expertise in these areas.

Shadowing the patient journey

While the above exercise is a useful introduction to the breadth of outpatient services, the best way for medical students and junior doctors to understand how these services work is to spend time with different people in each stage of the process. One way to achieve this is to ask any willing patients if they would be prepared to be 'shadowed' from the point they arrive in the clinic to the time they leave it. This can be an extremely illustrative experience and allows students to understand the pace and flow of how an outpatient service runs, and to hear firsthand the patients' views about their experiences. Additionally, spending time with non-clinical staff gives valuable insights into some of the systems and processes involved.

Managing Services in clinic

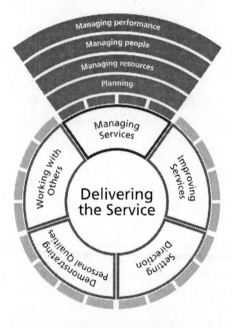

The MLCF describes how doctors demonstrate leadership by using their knowledge and influence to ensure resources are used efficiently and safely, to minimise waste and take action when resources are not being used efficiently and effectively.

Improving DNA rates

In the introduction we cited a figure of 6.7 million missed appointments (often referred to as 'Did Not Attend's [DNAs]) in the NHS in England over one year. The financial and logistical impact of this is huge. The Department of Health has estimated the cost of each missed appointment at around £100, which makes the annual cost to the NHS well over £600 million per year (over half of 1% of the total expenditure on health).

Image © 2010 NHS Institute and AoMRC

With these astronomical figures in mind, alongside the consideration of the personal inconvenience involved to patients, outpatient services are an excellent area for junior doctors to commit some 'project time' to work alongside managers, administrative and clerical staff, and senior colleagues to improve efficiency. The medical literature is a good starting point for ideas. There have been a number of initiatives around use of telephone or text message reminders in the days or hours prior to an appointment. A few key papers, including a Cochrane Systematic Review (2001, so with the dynamic nature of communications technology likely to be quickly out-of-date), are listed in the reference section (these include Reda and Makhoul, 2001; Roberts *et al.*, 2007; and Parikh *et al.*, 2010).

Activity capture

Another area crucial to efficiency and successfully managing resources is recording clinical activity. With the 'payment by results' tariff system described in the section above, every episode of activity that is not recorded appropriately costs the service provider (usually the department running the clinic) income. Improving activity capture needs the joint input of clinicians and administrators to develop thorough systems, but ones which have the least possible impact on clinical time. Clinical input to the design of these systems is crucial as much of the data collection involves what investigations, referrals and follow-up arrangements have been made.

Working alongside managers

If you have identified areas of inefficiency around appointment attendance, patient flows through clinics and the recording of your clinical activity, there are actions you can take to improve things. With the support of your supervising consultant, getting in touch with the service manager responsible for the outpatients service you work in to discuss some of these issues is a useful starting point. The vast majority of service managers will be delighted to hear from junior doctors and will be keen to gain their clinical insights. Although managers at this level may vary hugely in terms of experience, many will have a very similar number of years of healthcare experience to a doctor part-way through their postgraduate training, and there can be great synergy from managers and trainees working together on this sort of work.

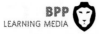

Undertaking projects like these presents a fantastic opportunity for both managers and junior doctors to learn from each other and develop a greater understanding of each other's perspectives, with the common aim of delivering high quality patient care. There is a more detailed description of this idea around 'paired-learning' in Chapter 11.

Improving Services in clinic

The earlier sections in this chapter have highlighted some of the key roles involved in running clinics and outpatient services. When considering how to improve services these same people are going to be important colleagues to engage in discussing any of your ideas for improvement. Another crucial group from which to seek input are patients and their carers.

Patient and carer feedback

Within the Improving Services domain, the MLCF describes how doctors show leadership by critically evaluating. This means thinking analytically and conceptually to identify where services can be improved, either through working individually or as part of a team. An important aspect of this includes obtaining and acting on patient, carer and service user feedback and experiences. Within the private sector innovative approaches to 'customer care' have been developed over many decades, but with only a few honourable exceptions, healthcare providers have been woefully slow to work in this area. Clearly patients are not 'customers' in the retail sense of the word, but the businesses who have spent huge resources in developing their understanding of their customers'

Image © 2010 NHS Institute and AoMRC

preferences have great expertise in this area; there is much we can learn from them which applies to our own services. Think about Exercise 5.2, a scenario about using patient and carer input to improve services:

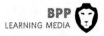

Exercise 5.2   Scenario

Mr B is an orthopedic registrar who does much of his out-patient work within fracture clinic. He has been asked by his consultant to work with the sister in fracture clinic to develop a mechanism for obtaining patient and carer feedback on their experiences. The team are hoping to expand the services they offer by bringing in more physiotherapist and occupational therapist input, but at the moment this has been put on hold. Mr B's consultant feels that this expansion is an important part of offering a holistic multi-professional service and wants to get the views of patients and carers to see whether they would support the ideas behind developing this new service.

- What tools or techniques could Mr B and colleagues use to obtain these views?
- How might they be able to use these views to bolster their case for expansion of the service?
- How can the learning from patient and carer views be disseminated to the wider clinical and management teams?

Summary of issues

There are increasing numbers of survey tools and other techniques to obtain the 'user view' of healthcare. Many of them now use advances in technology with web-based surveys and portable touch-screen devices as a way of getting feedback that can be instantaneously collated and disseminated. This approach is an excellent way to get real-time information, and once it is set up usually requires minimal resources to maintain, but there are two main disadvantages to consider. First, much of the information from these types of surveys tends to be ratings where patients are asked to give a score (eg out of 5) for different aspects of the service. While this enables a service provider to compare scores in different timeframes or across different areas of their service, it does not give descriptive information which can feed into improvement planning. The other disadvantage of these techniques of information collection is that, unless they are considered very carefully, they can preclude feedback from patients in certain vulnerable groups (eg people who cannot read English, people who do not understand the basics of touching a screen to give answers and people with learning difficulties and other disabilities).

Qualitative feedback from patients

Both of these disadvantages can be countered by taking a more qualitative approach to obtaining feedback from patients and their carers. This requires different techniques such as interviews, focus groups or comment cards, where instructions can be given in whatever language is understood by the patient. Although the feedback and learning from these methods is potentially richer, they are much more resource-heavy in terms of capturing and analysing the feedback. Many healthcare providers are starting to use a combination of quantitative and qualitative approaches to both track and learn from their patients' experiences. Independent organisations like the Picker Institute (http://pickerinstitute.org), who are focused on advancing the principles of patient-centred care, have developed a number of different tools which healthcare providers can use.

Disseminating the learning from patient feedback

One principle often missed in healthcare organisations is having a clear strategy to disseminate the learning from the patient views that are obtained. Unless there are ways in which the feedback loop is completed so that the lessons learned can be implemented, there is little point in collecting the feedback in the first place (see Figure 5.1).

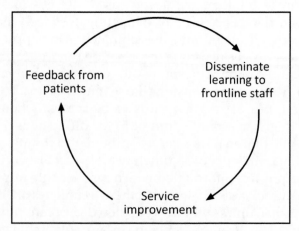

Figure 5.1 Learning from feedback

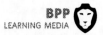

It is crucial that this information reaches the people delivering the frontline services, as they are the people who are often in the strongest position to act on it. Too often, feedback sits on the desks of senior managers and doctors without being effectively disseminated, discussed and reflected upon with the rest of the team. This is an important area that doctors in training in any department can contribute to. They should be encouraged to ask senior colleagues about their department's strategy for obtaining patient experience feedback. They can contribute to the process by thinking about the ways they may be able to support the dissemination and learning of this feedback, and therefore help influence improvements for patients.

Setting Direction in clinic

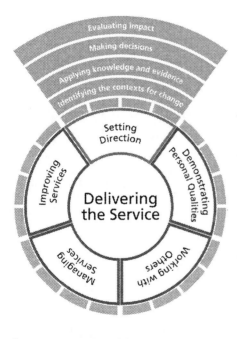

In the section on 'Setting Direction on the wards' in Chapter 4, we discussed integrated care pathways and the move towards healthcare being delivered in a much more cohesive way across the traditional primary-secondary care divide. Non-urgent, specialist, clinic-based work is an area where many healthcare providers are looking at more innovative ways to deliver services outside the traditional outpatients setting. One of the ideas you may have picked up from the literature about missed appointments is that there is good evidence to suggest a reasonable number of these occur because patients do not want to come into the hospital. It may be due to the logistics of travelling in, or because of memories that it brings back (of an earlier episode of illness for them or a family member), or for any number of other reasons. This is a particular problem with certain groups of the population ie young men, who are often cited as being poor at engaging with health services.

When working in an outpatient setting it is worth considering in more detail which groups of patients are least likely to engage with the services your department is offering. Are there approaches you could take to improve the situation? Exercise 5.3 below further explores this issue.

 Exercise 5.3   **Scenario**

Dr D is a Specialty Trainee in Genito-Urinary Medicine. The majority of her work is within the sexual health clinic based in the main hospital of the largest town in the region. The team she works with is aware of data that shows a high DNA rate for follow-up appointments. The feedback from local GP practices is that patients are reluctant to attend a sexual health clinic that is based in the hospital outpatient building. Dr D's educational supervisor has been asked to lead on developing a proposal to reconfigure the service so that it is more integrated with primary care. He has asked Dr D to help him lead this project.

- How might Dr D and her supervisor go about reconfiguring the service to address these issues?
- From where might they obtain information that they could use to develop their plans?
- Who might they need to talk with to discuss their proposals?
- How might they go about evaluating the impact of their proposed changes?

Summary of issues

There are many potential answers to this exercise and this type of project is likely to take many months to develop. Some of the key ideas you may have considered might be to consult with colleagues, work alongside local GPs and other primary care health workers, use patient experience feedback and use patient activity data. You may also have started to think about how your evaluation strategy might work. All of the ideas and concepts behind this exercise, and others like it, are highly accessible to bright and enthusiastic doctors in training, who are eager to gain experience in developing services for patients.

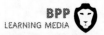

Departments with a strong training ethos should be seeking out these types of activities, and supporting and encouraging their junior doctors to contribute to them.

Summary

A huge amount of healthcare is delivered within clinics and outpatient services, therefore they provide an important arena for trainees and medical students to develop leadership competencies. This means developing an understanding of the complexity of healthcare systems, thinking about ways in which patient feedback can be used to influence change and participating in quality improvement projects. All of this is underpinned by the need to work as part of a team that is wholeheartedly focused on improving patient care.

 Three things to try

1. Explore how your department obtains feedback from patients – is there anything you could do to help disseminate the learning from this feedback amongst the clinical teams?
2. Find out what the DNA rates are for the clinics that you attend – are there any interventions you could try out to improve patient attendance at appointments?
3. Organise a time to meet with one of the managers in your department to find out more about their work – are there any projects you could work together on?

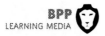

References

Bracken D *et al.* (1997) *Should 360-degree feedback be used only for developmental purposes?* Greensboro, NC: Center for Creative Leadership.

Campbell J *et al.* Validation of a multi-source feedback tool for use in general practice. *Education for Primary Care* 2010; 21: 165–179.

Department of Health. European Working Time Directive. [Online] Available at http://webarchive.nationalarchives.gov.uk/+/www.dh.gov.uk/en/Managingyourorganisation/Workforce/Workforceplanninganddevelopment/Europeanworkingtimedirective/DH_415 [Accessed 17/10/11].

Lelliott P *et al.* Questionnaires for 360-degree assessment of consultant psychiatrists: development and psychometric properties. *The British Journal of Psychiatry* 2008; 193(2): 156–160.

Parikh A *et al.* The effectiveness of outpatient appointment reminder systems in reducing no-show rates. *The American Journal of Medicine* 2010; 123(6): 542–548.

Reda S and Makhoul S. Prompts to encourage appointment attendance for people with serious mental illness. *Cochrane Database of Systematic Reviews* 2001: (2), CD002085. [Online] Available at http://www2.cochrane.org/reviews/ [Accessed 17/10/11].

Roberts N, Meade K and Partridge M. The effect of telephone reminders on attendance in respiratory outpatient clinics. *Journal of Health Services Research & Policy* 2007; 12(2): 69–72.

The NHS Information Centre. Provisional Monthly Hospital Episode Statistics for Admitted patient care, outpatient and Accident & Emergency data, April 2010. [Online] Available at www.ic.nhs.uk/pubs/provisionalmonthlyhes [Accessed 17/10/11].

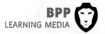

Chapter 6

Leadership Learning in Handover

Bob Klaber

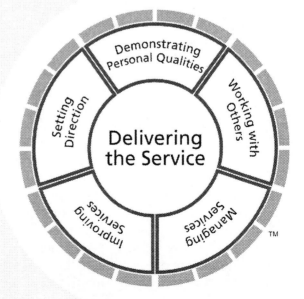

Chapter 6

Leadership Learning in Handover

 Chapter overview

This chapter examines the opportunities for leadership learning in handover, and explores a number of key concepts including:

- Learning and developing handover skills
- Leading handover
- Developing objectives and standards for handover
- Governance issues around using handover sheets
- Improving efficiency in meetings through the idea of a 'dollar clock'
- The role of junior doctors as handover 'experts'

 This chapter also looks at practical tools and techniques which can be used to support learning in and around handover. These include:

- Structured frameworks (such as Situation-Background-Assessment-Recommendation [SBAR]) to support handover
- Techniques for evaluating outcomes from handover

Introduction

Handover can be defined as 'the transfer of professional responsibility and accountability for some or all aspects of care for a patient, or group of patients, to another person or professional group on a temporary or permanent basis' (National Patient Safety Agency, 2004). Handing over responsibility for medical patients has always been part of medical practice, but formal handovers have increased in importance since the transition from 'on-calls' to predominately 'full-shift' working, in line with the implementation of the European Working Time Directive (Department of Health) in 2004. Departments responsible for acute patient care have had to incorporate two or three handover sessions into every day to ensure the incoming medical team understand patient problems and management plans. The vast majority of acute patient handover is done by junior members of the medical team, with varying degrees of senior supervision. Other departments with a less acute focus have also developed mechanisms to ensure the safe handover of patient care from one professional to another.

With this exponential increase in handover activity, clinicians have had to rapidly develop skills in handing over patients. These skills include the ability to summarise, prioritise, foresee potential problems and develop clear action plans for the team. Despite this, many healthcare providers fail to recognise that handover is a high risk area and so have done little to induce or train junior doctors in handover skills. The research literature around handover (or 'handoff' as it is called in some parts of the world) is growing. This includes a number of studies that illustrate that the quality of handover is often poor (ie Sabir *et al.*, 2006; Roughton and Severs, 1996). However, developing an understanding of how mistakes in handover might lead to serious failures can jump-start initiatives to improve patient safety.

Most of the early innovations around handover have been developed with help from outside medicine, for example using expertise from space, aviation, motor-racing and nuclear industries (Catchpole *et al.*, 2007; Catchpole *et al.*, 2010; and Patterson *et al.*, 2004). There are now increasing numbers of doctors starting to apply quality improvement methods to the handover processes in their place of work. This chapter aims to encourage junior doctors and medical students to reflect on their handover experiences to date, and to think about ways they can influence improvements on how handovers are run in their department.

Demonstrating Personal Qualities in handover

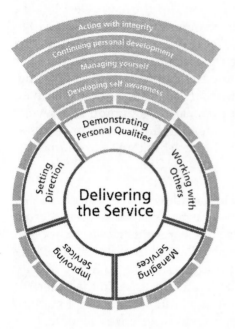

As described in earlier chapters the core aspects of this domain focus on self awareness and personal development. Up until the beginning of the 21st century there were very few areas of medicine where doctors practised regular handover of patients. The long working hours and on-call structures meant that, although the junior doctors may have been exhausted, there was strong continuity of care. As is evidenced by the medical literature, almost all of the historical work and expertise on handover had been nurse-led, as nurses sought to find ways to optimally handover patients to their colleague who was taking on the next shift. As a result there has been very little formal training available to doctors about handover. In many cases senior consultants and trainers, who have such depth of experience in so many areas, are themselves relatively inexperienced at running successful handovers. These are undoubtedly skills that can be learned.

Learning and developing handover skills

Working with Colin Macdougall, a paediatrician colleague, Bob Klaber undertook a project to consider the different ways of maximising learning opportunities in handover (Klaber and Macdougall, 2009). Alongside a review of the best available evidence, many of the ideas proposed were generated from working with a group of approximately 90 paediatricians with particular experience and interest in medical education. The results showed that in order for handover to be as safe as it possibly can be, the following seven ideas need to be considered:

Image © 2010 NHS Institute and AoMRC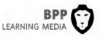

1. Departments need to have a consistent approach that handover is important and valued.
2. A clear structure is needed to reflect the local purposes of different handovers.
3. Trainees come with a variety of experiences that could help or hinder local practice – capturing experiences they bring from previous jobs can be a valuable source of new ideas.
4. Handover skills need to be learned and improved during training and beyond.
5. There are many different opportunities for trainees to learn about clinical or systems-based issues in handover but utilising these takes effort and planning.
6. There needs to be careful thought about how to give feedback during or around handover.
7. If handover is to improve, this needs ongoing reflection, audit and perhaps assessment.

(Klaber and Macdougall, 2009)

Underpinning all of this is for individual students and doctors to be given opportunities to learn and develop their handover skills. Handover is starting to be incorporated into both undergraduate and postgraduate curricula and some medical schools, Deaneries and Trusts are developing training programmes to support the development of these competencies. The development of work-place based assessments (WPBAs) such as case-based discussions (CbDs) offer opportunities for these educational initiatives to be underpinned by assessment. In addition to any formal strategies for 'handover learning', departments need to work hard to support a culture of feedback and personal development around handover.

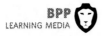

Working with Others in handover

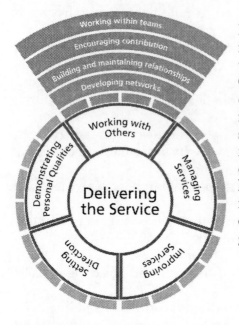

Excellent teamworking is essential for handover to be successful and safe. On occasions there may be consultant or senior nursing input although most shift-to-shift patient handovers are run amongst a group of junior doctors. Trainees running handover need to develop skills in prioritisation and delegation of tasks. An example of this is given in Exercise 6.1.

 ### Exercise 6.1   Scenario

Dr Q is a paediatric registrar who is running the morning handover. The team receiving handover with her are a Foundation Year doctor, a Year 3 specialty trainee and the ward sister. A medical student is also present. The team has been given the handover sheet below, which the Year 2 specialty trainee on-call overnight had prepared:

             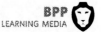

Exercise 6.1 *(Continued)*   **Scenario**

Name	Age	Duration of admission	Presenting complaint/ diagnosis	Results of investigations	Actions completed to date
John	1 yr	10 hours	Fracture of right femur. Fell from sofa.		On orthopedic theatre list for today
Sara	12 yrs	3 days	Diabetes. Frequent admissions with DKA. Threatening to self-discharge from the ward.	HBA1c 9.7%	On revised insulin regimen
Rose	10 yrs	12 hours	Right iliac fossa pain. Second admission with similar symptoms.	FBC and CRP normal	Surgical review awaited
Jamila	7 yrs	4 days	Right sided pneumonia with pleural effusion.	CRP 233, CXR shows a large effusion	Ultrasound of chest awaited
Asif	6 days	6 hours	Admitted with fever of 39.1°C. Unsettled and off feeding. No clear focus found.	Hb 12.1, WBC 14.6, N 11.2, Plt 333. CRP 26 Awaiting urine	Being observed. Not had any antibiotics
Aman	4 yrs	1 day	D&V. On vacation from Malawi. Parents keen to be discharged as soon as possible.	Stool cultures negative so far	Oral rehydration
Daisy	7 yrs	1 day	Receiving chemotherapy for Stage 4 neuroblastoma. Febrile neutropenia.	FBC – Hb 7.9, WBC 0.6, N 0.0, Plt 102, CRP < 5	On first line IV antibiotics

- How should Dr Q go about prioritising the tasks for the day?
- How could she allocate different tasks to each of the team members in order to get the team working as effectively as possible?

Summary of issues

Unless you have a reasonable knowledge of paediatrics it would be unfair to expect you to identify the nuances of each of the cases presented. Essentially the handover sheet represents a potentially septic baby, a child protection concern and a number of other medical, social and bed-management issues that need addressing with different levels of urgency. However, as well as a requirement for medical knowledge to identify clinical problems, this exercise has highlighted that successful handover needs to incorporate prioritisation, delegation of tasks and strong team-working.

Leading handover

In order to achieve these elements there needs to be clarity about who is 'leading' or 'chairing' each handover. It may be that a department feels this is best done by the attending consultant; another may feel this role should be fulfilled by the registrar at the end of their shift. If senior clinicians take on this role there need to be opportunities for junior members of the team to gain experience in chairing handovers. They also need to be given feedback that supports them in developing these key skills. Finally, there needs to be clarity about who is taking on this lead role in each handover that occurs. This may be simply achieved through a brief discussion, or can be more visually highlighted by the person chairing the handover sitting on a different coloured chair. While this may seem the sort of setup more likely to be found at a children's birthday party, any innovation that gives clarity to the purpose and direction of handover is likely to result in more effective team-working and hence safer handover.

The 'dollar clock'

Another handover issue, and one that applies to all meetings, is to consider whether everyone who is present really needs to be there, either for the safe transfer of information or for their own learning. Large meetings that continue for hours and hours need to be recognised as expensive in terms of using up the time of large numbers of people. One way to focus minds on this is through the idea of a 'dollar clock'.

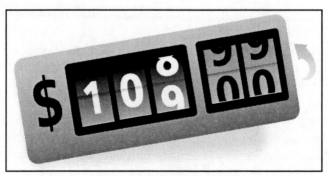

Figure 6.1 A 'dollar clock'

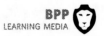

Imagine a clock or counter into which everyone in the meeting types in their nominal hourly rate – putting this into dollars gives it a slightly abstract feel but still focuses the mind. When the meeting begins the counter starts and the cost rises as every minute passes. The more people present, the quicker the costs escalate. In many ways, briefly highlighting this imaginary exercise to handover participants is all that needs to happen, but it would be eminently possible to build a program on a smartphone or other portable computer that could actually give a visual display.

Managing Services in handover

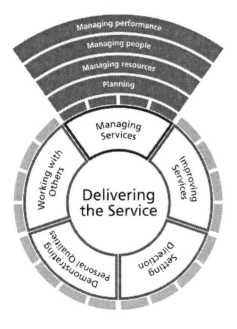

Safe and efficient handover needs to be thought of as a fundamental cornerstone to successfully managing inpatient and emergency services. There are also examples where the care of chronic patients is highly dependent on effective handover of information and responsibility. Three of the elements that form the *Managing Services* domain in the MLCF focus on managing people, managing performance and managing resources, and an appreciation of all of these competencies is needed to run handover effectively.

Objectives and standards for handover

The starting point for successful handover in any department is having real clarity of purpose, and this needs to come from the senior clinicians. Each handover at the different times of the day or week should have unambiguous objectives so that all participants are focused on what needs to be achieved. Departments should have standards that, having been spelled out during induction at the start of their post, give clarity to how participants in handover are expected to work. This should lead to clear ground rules covering issues such as time-keeping, different roles, use of typed handover sheets and structure. Issues concerning roles were discussed in the 'Working with Others' section above, and ideas involving written sheets and handover structure are discussed below.

Handover sheets

In the early days of medical handover, written handover sheets were considered an unnecessary risk to patient confidentiality. However, there is now a small body of evidence in the medical literature that suggests that using typed handover sheets supports the retention of key knowledge (Bhabra *et al.*, 2007; Ferran *et al.*, 2008). The majority of departments now use a system of typed handover sheets, although some are developing initiatives to use web-based systems linked to electronic patient records or other types of electronic device (Van Eaton *et al.*, 2005; Raptis *et al.*, 2009). There are interesting governance issues regarding written handover sheets, and it seems prudent that each version of the handover sheet (ie each time it is updated) is saved under a different file name in a password protected, encrypted folder within the Trust's computer network. In this way there is a record that can be reviewed and retrospectively audited if needed. There are simple ways to encourage safe disposal of the handover sheets; asking everyone to write their name on the top of the sheet and placing a confidential waste bin in the room where handover takes place are both effective strategies.

Structuring handover

Ideas involving giving handover a structure or communication framework are increasing within the medical literature. Of these, the most widely used is the Situation-Background-Assessment-Recommendation (SBAR) framework, originally used by the military and aviation industries and adapted for use in healthcare by Dr M Leonard and colleagues from Kaiser Permanente in Colorado, USA (Institute for Healthcare Improvement). They describe the technique below:

> *The SBAR (Situation-Background-Assessment-Recommendation) technique provides a framework for communication between members of the health care team about a patient's condition. SBAR*

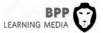

is an easy-to-remember, concrete mechanism useful for framing any conversations, especially critical ones, requiring a clinician's immediate attention and action. It allows for an easy and focused way to set expectations for what will be communicated and how between members of the team, which is essential for developing teamwork and fostering a culture of patient safety.

(Institute for Healthcare Improvement, 2005)

Leonard had previously demonstrated the positive impact on patient safety of a standardised communication process within Kaiser Permanente, a non-profit American healthcare system providing care for 8.3 million patients (Leonard *et al.*, 2004). SBAR has been used worldwide in a wide range of situations, and has been particularly helpful in giving junior staff a mechanism, which they know is embedded in the culture of their organisation, to highlight patient safety issues to senior colleagues (Featherstone, 2005). It has also been used in a number of organisations as a structure for the handover of patients at the end of a shift. An example of how SBAR can be used in this way is given in Table 6.1.

Situation
• Identify the patient by name and which clinical area they are in
• Give additional information that might help with prioritisation

Background
• Give the patient's reason for admission and date of admission
• Explain the significant medical history, examination findings, investigations, working diagnosis and management plan to date
• Describe any key aspects of the patient's background

Assessment
• Give the latest clinical observations (ideally as a trend)
• Describe your clinical impression and/or concerns

Recommendation
• Explain what you need – be specific about the request and timeframe
• Make suggestions
• Clarify expectations

Table 6.1 How SBAR can be used

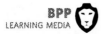

More important than the specifics of this particular tool is the recognition that giving handover a clarity of purpose, expected standards and a structure are important steps towards ensuring it is both safer and more efficient.

Improving Services in handover

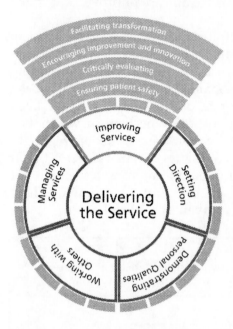

As detailed in the MLCF, *Improving Services* describes a process of facilitating transformation to deliver safe, innovative, high quality care to patients. In the section above on 'Managing Services in handover' we discussed different ideas around strategies to ensure that handover is as safe as possible. These are by no means exhaustive, and while one of them might work well in one particular handover environment, others may not.

Junior doctors improving handover

As mentioned in the introduction, in many ways junior doctors are the experts in handover. The nature of their shifts means they spend a significant part of their working week in handover, and their frequently rotating posts give them a range of handover experiences from different healthcare organisations across their region. This puts them in a strong position to recognise the risks around handover and also to design, implement and evaluate improvements to the handovers they participate in. To achieve this they need enthusiasm, determination and the support and supervision of senior colleagues to make change happen.

Exercise 6.2   Scenario

Dr H is a surgical trainee who has just rotated into a new post in a large teaching hospital. He is concerned that the handover of patients from the overnight team to the different surgical specialties is fairly haphazard. Information is meant to be handed over face-to-face, but in reality this often happens over the phone and there is no written handover sheet to support the process. There have been two recent occasions where theatre lists were delayed because the appropriate information had not been handed over to the relevant team at the beginning of the day. He has experienced a number of different handover arrangements in his placements to date and is keen to make some improvements to the current setup to make it safer and more efficient.

- What steps should Dr H take in planning changes to the surgical handover?
- Who should he talk to about his proposals?
- What implementation strategies are most likely to be successful?
- How will he know if he has been successful in making improvements to the current system?

Summary of issues

As with any improvement project, there are a number of important steps that Dr H will need to undertake. Improving handover requires looking at how your handover currently runs, identifying aspects that are not as strong as they could be and then going through design, planning and implementation stages. Identifying the current difficulties may be very clear to everyone involved, but some situations may need an audit of current practice to highlight the areas of concern. There may be guidelines from national bodies (such as the Royal College of Surgeons), or evidence in the literature that highlights 'best practice' from which a local guideline can be derived. Consulting with key people who are likely to have opinions and influence over the proposals (often called 'stakeholders') is important. The effort put in talking to colleagues to explain what you are trying to achieve and listening to their views is rarely wasted. It is worth thinking about the timing of implementation of any project like this; there are sometimes advantages in implementing a new initiative as a group of new junior doctors come into the department. In other situations it may be best to pilot the project

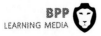

with a small group of colleagues who you have been working with for a period of time, and who can act as 'critical friends'.

Setting Direction in handover

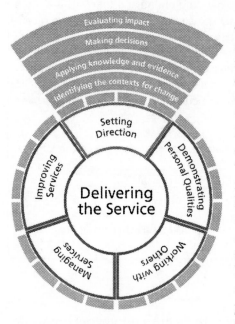

One of the most important aspects of implementing an improvement project and evaluating the impact of the change is often the piece of the jigsaw that is overlooked. In the *Setting Direction* domain of the MLCF, the 'evaluating impact' element refers to doctors showing leadership through measuring and evaluating outcomes, and formally and informally disseminating good practice. Developing an evaluation strategy should be part of the *planning* process of any type of service improvement project and not just left as an afterthought. Before any idea can be given approval for wider implementation there needs to be a degree of clarity, even if it is not 'Grade A evidence', of its impact.

Evaluating the impact of improvement projects

Evaluations can take a wide range of forms, ranging from informal questioning of participants, up to larger scale audits and external observations of behaviour. The strategy you choose for your project will depend on the questions you are hoping to answer. Evaluating the impact of any improvement plan that you might have for your department's handover sessions can also take a number of forms (Jeffcott *et al.*, 2009). These include a:

*   Patient safety focus – in this scenario you may want to audit different markers of safe/unsafe care. These may include auditing the impact on clinical incident reports relating to

Image © 2010 NHS Institute and AoMRC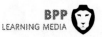

miscommunication, or using a ward-round scoring system to assess what percentage of key information was handed on to the incoming team.

- Teamworking focus – in this scenario you may want to look at ways to examine team behaviours in handover. This can be done using video-based scoring systems or through asking an external observer (a role that could definitely be undertaken by a medical student) to observe and map the conversations and interactions that occur.
- Participant experience focus – in this scenario you may want to use more qualitative approaches, such as semi-structured interviews or focus groups, to get participants' views of the impact of your intervention. Another method is to use 'satisfaction score' surveys.

In addition to the evaluation itself there needs to be a strategy to feedback the information and learning that has been gained, so that the intervention can be improved even further.

Summary

Handover has become fundamental to the successful delivery of safe patient care, and is an integral part of the vast majority of departments in which junior doctors and medical students are training. As well as gaining knowledge from clinical discussions, handover offers an excellent opportunity to develop leadership skills. This means thinking about how teams function at their best and using evidence to inform improvements, implement change and evaluate the impact. This is undoubtedly a clinical area where trainees can have a huge impact on improving patient care.

Three things to try

1. Have a discussion with colleagues about setting explicit objectives and standards for each of the clinical handovers that occur in your department each week.
2. Experiment with using a structured framework (such as SBAR) to support the handover of patients.
3. Explore whether there are any outcome measures that you could use to assess how safe and effective your handovers are? (The references section should help with this.)

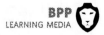

References

Bhabra G *et al*. An experimental comparison of handover methods. *Annals of the Royal College of Surgeons of England* 2007; 89(3): 298–300.

Catchpole K *et al*. Patient handover from surgery to intensive care: using Formula 1 pit-stop and aviation models to improve safety and quality. *Pediatric Anesthesia* 2007; 17(5): 470–478.

Catchpole K *et al*. Patient handovers within the hospital: translating knowledge from motor racing to healthcare. *Quality & Safety in Health Care* 2010; 19(4): 318–322.

Department of Health. European Working Time Directive. [Online] Available at http://webarchive.nationalarchives.gov.uk/+/ www.dh.gov.uk/en/Managingyourorganisation/Workforce/ Workforceplanninganddevelopment/Europeanworkingtimedirective/ DH_415 [Accessed 17/10/11].

Featherstone D. Interview with Frances A Griffin, Institute for Healthcare Improvement. *J Nurs Care Qual* 2005; 20(4): 369–372.

Ferran NA, Metcalfe AJ and O'Doherty D. Standardised proformas improve patient handover: Audit of trauma handover practice. *Patient Safety in Surgery* 2008; 2: 24.

Institute for Healthcare Improvement (2005) *SBAR technique for communication: a situational briefing model*. [Online] Available at www.ihi.org/IHI/Topics/PatientSafety/SafetyGeneral/Tools/ SBARTechniqueforCommunicationASituationalBriefingModel.htm [Accessed 17/10/11].

Jeffcott SA *et al*. Improving measurement in clinical handover. *Quality & Safety in Health Care* 2009; 18(4): 272–277.

Klaber RE and Macdougall CF. Maximising learning opportunities in handover. *Archives of Disease in Childhood. Education and Practice Edition* 2009; 94(4): 118–122.

Leonard M, Graham S and Bonacum D. The human factor: the critical importance of effective teamwork and communication in providing safe care. *Quality & Safety in Health Care* 2004; 13 Suppl 1: 85–90.

NPSA (2004) *Safe Handover: Safe Patients*. [Online] Available at www.bma. org.uk/images/safehandover_tcm41-20983.pdf [Accessed 17/10/11].

Patterson ES *et al*. Handoff strategies in settings with high consequences for failure: lessons for health care operations. *Int J Qual Health Care* 2004; 16(2): 125–132.

Raptis DA *et al*. Electronic software significantly improves quality of handover in a London teaching hospital. *Health Informatics Journal* 2009; 15(3): 191–198.

Roughton VJ and Severs MP. The junior doctor handover: current practices and future expectations. *Journal of the Royal College of Physicians of London* 1996; 30(3): 213–214.

Sabir N, Yentis SM and Holdcroft A. A national survey of obstetric anaesthetic handovers. *Anaesthesia* 2006; 61(4): 376–380.

Van Eaton EG *et al*. A randomized, controlled trial evaluating the impact of a computerized rounding and sign-out system on continuity of care and resident work hours. *Journal of the American College of Surgeons* 2005; 200(4): 538–545.

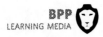

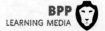

Chapter 7

Leadership Learning in the Emergency Department

Francesca Cleugh & Bob Klaber

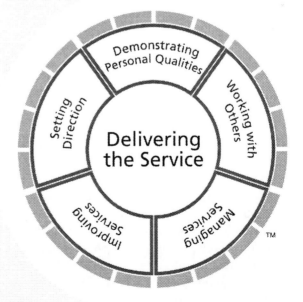

Leadership Learning in the Emergency Department

 Chapter overview

This chapter examines the opportunities for leadership learning in the Emergency Department, and explores a number of key concepts including:

- The impact of stress on doctors
- Teamworking
- Learning through shadowing
- Process targets (eg the four-hour wait)
- Local improvement initiatives
- Innovation
- Lean thinking
- Experience-based design
- Applying evidence to improve services

 This chapter also looks at practical tools and techniques which can be used to support learning. These include:

- Strategies to manage stress
- Mentoring
- Debrief
- Board rounds, and a handover tool to support Emergency Department work
- BestBETS evidence-based reviews

Introduction

Developing skills to assess and manage patients in an emergency care setting is a core part of learning for all medical students and junior doctors. Even if a doctor's career path takes them away from the Emergency Department (ED) and other unscheduled care environments, their patients, whether they are children, the elderly or people with mental health issues, will continue to experience healthcare in these settings. Understanding the impact on patients of acute illness, and their interactions with the healthcare system that result, is key for all doctors and health professionals. Emergency Departments (also known as 'Accident & Emergency'

or 'A&E' to much of the UK population) are often extremely busy areas where, due to the unpredictable nature of the numbers of patients and their different problems, there are huge complexities that need to be taken into account to run safe, high quality and efficient services.

The large throughput of patients, the clinical variety, the diverse workforce, the immediate management of critical illness and trauma, the patient flow outcome measurements (such as the four-hour wait target) and the interactions with both primary care and specialty teams provide many challenges and stimulating experiences. Working as part of a team within these complexities offers junior doctors an excellent opportunity to develop many different leadership competencies across all five domains of the MLCF. Many of the ideas and concepts that we will discuss are also very applicable to other clinical areas. This chapter will support medical students, junior doctors and those in a training role to explore opportunities for learning and improvement within emergency and urgent care settings.

Demonstrating Personal Qualities in the Emergency Department

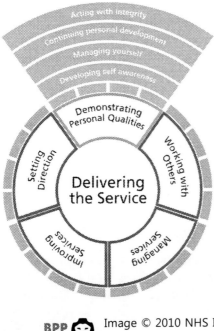

The previous chapters, have focused on leadership learning on the wards, in clinic settings, and in handover. There has been a strong focus on ideas concerning self-awareness, seeking feedback and continuing professional development. While there are many opportunities for students and trainees working in emergency care settings to develop experiences in these areas, this chapter will focus on the third of the four elements in the *Demonstrating Personal Qualities* domain.

This element is titled 'managing yourself'. The MLCF explains that doctors show leadership through managing themselves: fulfilling commitments, organising and managing themselves (without compromising their own health) while taking account of the needs and priorities of others. This requires doctors to recognise and manage the impact of their emotions on their own behaviour, and consider how this may impact on others around them.

Stress in doctors: the wider impact

Many doctors will put a huge amount of thought and energy into the care they provide for their patients, and in the support they offer their colleagues, but they are often not very good at looking after themselves (Firth-Cozens, 2003). From both cross-sectional and longitudinal studies, we know the proportion of doctors and other health professionals showing above-threshold levels of stress has stayed relatively constant at approximately 28%, compared with about 18% in the general working population (Wall *et al.*, 1997; Firth-Cozens, 1999). Stress is a difficult concept to define, but perhaps the definition most applicable to medicine comes from the mid-1980s: when *'pressure exceeds one's perceived ability to cope'* (Lazarus & Folkman, 1984). Factors such as excessive workloads, dealing with patients' suffering, and living with one's own mistakes or fear of them, are often cited as major contributers to stress in doctors. This can be exacerbated by uncertainties around career progression, a lack of professional support, and inadequate training (particularly in areas such as communication skills, teamworking, leadership and management) (Iversen *et al.*, 2009). Stress is important as it can lead to more serious disorders such as anxiety disorder, depression and/or alcohol and drug-dependence in doctors. It is also very important for patients; studies suggest that doctors are more likely to make errors and perform sub-optimally if they are stressed. One case-control study found that the introduction of stress management courses to 22 hospitals was associated with a substantial reduction in the rate of negligence and malpractice claims as compared with the control hospitals (Jones *et al.*, 1988).

Developing strategies to manage stress

There is a huge amount in the medical literature about preventing stress-related disorders in doctors, although as highlighted by a recent systematic review (McCray *et al.*, 2008), where only very few studies met the inclusion criteria, evidence for any particular interventions is very light. In their excellent review *How to handle stress and look after your mental health* Iverson and colleagues suggest a number of ideas and methods that may help to prevent stress-related disorders in junior doctors (Iversen *et al.*, 2009). Some of the points are based on the small evidence-base that exists while others are ideas that come from the authors. A few of the key suggestions are detailed below:

- Find regular times for 'self-care' (eg sport or exercise, meditation or reading a non-medical book)
- Find a mentor, ideally someone 'offline', who you do not directly work with
- Become more reflective: find time to acknowledge your emotions
- Find time for your family and friends
- Reflect on your own personal values then give these a renewed focus
- Support your own development of any specific skills that might help (eg through specific reading or attending a course)

It is worth getting a copy of the original publication (Iversen *et al.*, 2009), especially as this review also has an extremely useful list of resources of where to find support if you need it. The British Medical Association (BMA) offers a number of different services to support doctors, and most Deaneries and medical schools will also have services or support networks for doctors who need help and advice.

Support from colleagues

Doctors working in the ED need to recognise and acknowledge how the pressures of their work can impact on their own health and wellbeing at different stages of their careers. Many departments have established mentoring schemes (often pairing up an experienced nurse with a junior doctor), or other initiatives where staff receive support from their colleagues. The aim is to provide individuals with the space and time to reflect on how a particular situation has affected their emotions. From a survey-based study of almost 200 emergency physicians in the USA, high levels of anxiety (caused by concern for bad outcomes) were the strongest predictor of

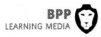

burnout (Kuhn *et al.*, 2009). The focus of many of the leadership competencies described in the MLCF are on teamworking and supporting colleagues, and these are hugely important factors in managing and supporting colleagues through periods of anxiety and self-doubt. Senior doctors have an overall responsibility for the welfare of their junior staff, but peer support amongst doctors and other health professionals working together in the ED can have a positive impact on managing stress.

Working with Others in the Emergency Department

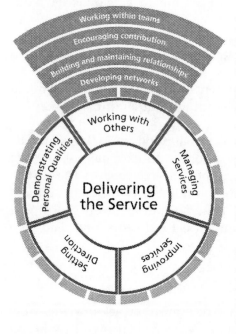

Health professionals working in emergency settings do so in a number of different teams. This may be the team of junior doctors at the same stage of training who make up a rota, the multiprofessional team who work in a particular area of the ED or the team of professionals who are working together through a particular shift. These different teams will encounter a wide range of challenges in their work, and their ability to work and learn together as a team is fundamental to successfully delivering high quality patient care.

Teamworking in a resuscitation

Perhaps the most illustrative example of teamworking comes from the resuscitation of a critically ill patient, although there are many other situations where the same principles apply. In order to have the greatest chance of being successful, a resuscitation requires a group of individual health professionals, each with their own area

Image © 2010 NHS Institute and AoMRC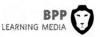

of skill and expertise, to work together as a team in a highly co-ordinated and efficient way. As well as the medical challenges of deciphering what has caused the problem and how it should be managed, the team has to cope with a significant emotional burden as well. Most obviously this is about very closely supporting the patient's family through everything that is happening, and in understanding that events like this can have a profound effect on the wellbeing of different individual members of the team. Recognising and addressing these issues in colleagues can be difficult, and is usually most successful in departments where there is a real ethos of team support. Achieving successful teamworking requires commitment, training and leadership (Lerner *et al.*, 2009). A strong team culture can be supported by pre-brief, focusing on clarification of roles and responsibilities, simulation-based training and debrief.

Debrief

Debrief enables individual members of the team to reflect on their own performance and to identify errors and successes. In addition, debrief encourages the team to come together to discuss and review team processes and interactions. This allows team members to have a stronger understanding of any issues that have been identified with the systems or processes the team is using. It also enables everyone to reflect together in developing a shared mental model of the team's performance. With this approach the team can come to a consensus of what methods or approaches did or did not work and decide on strategies to improve future performance. This provides a much more constructive approach than the traditional 'blame culture' where feedback is only ever negative. By using the debrief process to focus on *what* is right rather than *who* is right, teams can begin to identify and mitigate causes of error much more effectively. In their excellent review article on developing expert medical teams, Fernandez and colleagues make several suggestions for establishing debrief, using the evidence-base from the team training literature:

- Debrief should be diagnostic, to identify strengths and weaknesses and expose latent errors
- Debrief should be used to facilitate the development of strategies to mitigate future errors

- Training programmes should be designed to allow for the provision of *immediate* feedback
- Debrief should occur in a supportive environment focused on process improvement
- Debriefing facilitators should be appropriately trained and utilise evidence-based methodology
- Team leaders should become proficient in debriefing to facilitate the transfer of reflection to the clinical setting
- The content, timing, and frequency of debrief should directly relate to the learning objectives and level of the learner
- Credibility of feedback is crucial and can be enhanced with the use of video recordings or objective checklists

(Fernandez *et al.*, 2008; Salas *et al.*, 2008)

Although these criteria were developed in the context of team-training, which is likely to occur in a simulated format, you should be able to look through the suggestions for debrief above to see how they would apply to the example of a resuscitation team in an ED. The emphasis on a diagnostic approach, which is focused on strategies to mitigate future error and on process improvements, is crucial. If led by experienced trainers who are genuinely able to create a working atmosphere where all team members are comfortable giving each other feedback, then establishing a debriefing culture can have a significant impact on successfully delivering safe and high quality care.

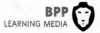

Managing Services in the Emergency Department

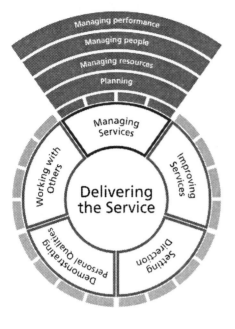

In 2009–2010, over 20 million people attended Emergency Departments in England (Department of Health, 2011). This is a rise of approximately 50% over the last 20 years. There are many factors contributing to the increase. In the UK, it is thought that changes to the GP out-of-hours contract in 2004 had a palpable impact. Additionally, increasing expectations of patients, demographic changes and organisational changes (that have caused confusion about how to access urgent care) have interplayed to put increasing pressure on Emergency Departments globally (Lowthian et al., 2010). Along with the rising pressure of workload there is also an expectation to perform well, and managing performance has become an integral part of providing emergency care. In this section we will look at some of the ways clinicians can rise to the challenge of improving the quality of services they deliver.

Learning through shadowing

Shadowing the ED Registrar is an invaluable way to learn how to adapt to the ever-changing flow through the ED. When allocated to be in charge of the department, their role is to work closely with the nurse in charge, co-ordinate the staff and skill-mix across the ED to ensure patients are seen efficiently and safely, no matter how busy the shift. They must know when to escalate issues to the consultant and liaise with the site manager to redistribute staff from other areas if necessary. An extreme example of this would be in the event of a major incident. Each hospital has a policy in place for how to co-ordinate a major incident. Reading through a local policy is a great way to learn what factors need to be considered, such as calling in off-duty staff, cancelling elective admissions and discharging patients to create bed space. Those involved in planning for major incidents take part in simulation table-top exercises, and these are the sort of opportunities that students and trainees can observe and be involved with. These simulated exercises are an outstanding opportunity to learn from the decision-making and prioritising of those commanding the situation.

Managing the workload: board rounds

Even without a major incident, a heaving waiting room, staff sick leave and a high volume of trauma calls can stretch a department to capacity. Good leadership from the doctors and nurses managing the department is imperative to ensure that safe and high quality care is delivered, no matter how stretched the department is. Communication between members of the ED team and specialties is paramount. Any doctor working within the department must be adaptative to different roles to be able to meet the varying demand of each shift. The team can maintain an overview of the workload through regular board rounds.

Managing the workload: flexible staffing levels

Research has shown that patterns of patient attendance, seemingly random, are actually largely predictable (Walley, 2003). However, different hospitals will experience different patterns, and understanding local variation is a vital part of staff rota design. In many regions the under-one age group most often present out of hours, at night time (Downing and Wilson, 2002) and therefore these departments should ensure there are experienced paediatric doctors on shift overnight, but in other areas this may be less of an issue. ED rotas are notoriously antisocial for doctors working them, but as you can see there is a strong rationale behind this. The experience that junior doctors have of working these rotas is an invaluable resource to the service managers and consultants, and in all departments the 'trainee voice' should strongly contribute to the process of rota design and implementation.

Handover

With the fluctuation in workload as well as regular board rounds, it is important that at shift changes, particularly between the registrars in charge of the department, handover is precise and comprehensive. Tools for optimising handover and opportunities for leadership learning within it are discussed in detail in Chapter 6. There are, however, some unique factors to the ED that need careful consideration. An illustrative example is described below.

Case study

In a busy central London teaching hospital, locally led research showed that information conveyed between shifts had wide variation. During semi-structured interviews, along with identifying discrepancies, team members contributed their views of best practice for pertinent information that should be handed over. A consensus list was compiled. From this a tool was created to facilitate the handover process. The 'ABC of Handover' is a crib sheet filled out at handover between each shift. It gives a clear overview of the department, raising any issues that need escalation and how this was done. Using the mnemonic ABCDE, there is space to record pertinent patient and operational issues such as volume and level of care of patients, staffing allocation and shortfalls, unforeseen or unplanned events and any problems with equipment or other specialties contributing to the department. Local research revealed that the implementation of this simple tool improved communication and ensured a safer handover between shifts (Farhan et al., 2010).

Process targets

Along with coping with the impact of increasing numbers of patients attending the ED, there is the pressure to perform well. The most high profile performance measure of recent years in the ED has been the four hour 'breach' target. In 2000 the Department of Health published *The NHS Plan* (Department of Health, 2000) which stated that by 2004, patients should spend no longer than four hours within the ED. The target was met with resistance, having been imposed with relatively little consultation of those on the frontline of emergency care (Mortimore and Cooper, 2007). In recognising the need for some patients to spend longer in the ED, certain exemptions were set but the original 90% target was increased to 98% in 2005. At the time, acute hospital trusts in the UK were subject to a number of other key targets, and were 'star-rated' on their performance of these. Getting a zero star rating put the future survival of the trust on the line. Gaining three stars brought with it 'earned autonomy' with less central monitoring and inspections, and more control over finances and resources (Department of Health, 2001). There were massive implications for a hospital trust if more than 2% of ED attendees breached the four hour target, and many junior doctors came under pressure from senior medical, nursing or management colleagues to make timely decisions and discharge patients as quickly as possible.

Gaming to meet targets

Most hospitals did well in meeting their targets and made a significant impact on the experiences of patients, but it is well acknowledged that some were doing so by what is known as 'gaming'. During weeks that were closely monitored, extra staff might have been brought in or patients were kept in the ambulance bay until the department had capacity to see them (Bevan and Hood, 2006). Indeed some clinicians have argued that quality of care was affected, with time pressures on staff hindering thorough history-taking or the resolution of complex or social issues. Approaching the breach time, rushed admission decisions were made, sometimes resulting in deterioration of patients in wards soon afterwards (Rawlinson, 2008) and perhaps in other cases unnecessary admissions. Critics argued that trusts were *'hitting the target, but missing the point'* (Bevan and Hood, 2006).

In the weeks after the formation of the coalition government in 2010, plans to move away from top-down process targets were announced (Department of Health, 2010). There was a stated aim to move towards targets and measures that were focused on patient outcomes and not solely on processes. The four hour target was relaxed to 95%, welcomed by the College of Emergency Medicine (CEM press release, June 2010). No-one would want to see a return to patients spending 12 hours on trolleys in corridors, and most staff feel that managing the majority of patients within the four hour window is a good thing (Mortimore and Cooper, 2007). The challenge now for clinicians working in EDs is to hit both 'the target' and 'the point'.

Local improvement initiatives

The focus is undoubtedly now on clinicians to provide innovative local initiatives that ensure quality patient care. The introduction of new roles, such as Advanced Nurse Practitioners and Emergency Nurse Practitioners, with increased autonomy to manage their own patients, takes pressure off busy wait times. Empowering the triage nurse to see and treat some attenders, and having senior decision-makers within the department at the busiest times, improves patient flow while also improving quality. Thinking about the design and layout of the department, changing the set up of dressing trolleys, or altering patient flows through minor areas can dramatically improve efficiency and safety.

The knowledge and experience of clinicians of all levels within a busy ED is an invaluable 'improvement' resource to tap into. Empowering the team to devise locally relevant ways to meet the four hour target and continually strive for improved quality is crucial. When you are working in the ED, take time to look at the systems and setup; think about ways to improve flow and share them with the rest of your clinical and management team. As the 'ABC of Handover' in the earlier case study has shown, collaborative working within a department can have an outstandingly positive impact on the quality of service patients receive.

Improving Services in the Emergency Department

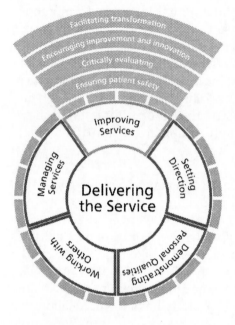

It is clear from just the few examples discussed so far that the ED is the perfect place to cultivate innovation and improvement.

Innovation

Innovation is taking something that already exists and making changes, often subtle, which make it work better in the current context. It does not have to be a completely new idea or invention (Plamping *et al.*, 2009). A fresh perspective is a key catalyst to creative and innovative thinking; this is where being a junior doctor, regularly moving between departments, opens up advantages. In their first few weeks, trainees who have just started within the department will notice glitches in the department's systems and processes. With the support of established senior colleagues, they can be encouraged to think about creative solutions before they become part of the status quo of the department. Doctors can demonstrate leadership by respectfully challenging the status quo. This may require courage and bravery, but undoubtedly the culture is slowly changing to facilitate and reward such thinking.

> ... *Strategies and processes alone are not sufficient to drive the degree of change we are seeking... the NHS should focus on tackling the behaviours and cultures in the system that stand in the way.*

> (David Nicholson CEO, National Health Service
> Annual Report, 2009)

Image © 2010 NHS Institute and AoMRC

The other clinical and non-clinical frontline staff, and of course patients, are another source of support and innovation. Most EDs have hundreds of patients each day, and staff from many different specialties will spend some time working there too. With their input and the right tools, innovative ideas can thrive. Two 'quality improvement' tools that work well in improving services in the ED are 'lean thinking' and 'experience-based design'. Both have been used in other industries for years, and as healthcare slowly catches up, their use has, in places, brought with it outstanding results (www.institute.nhs.uk).

Lean thinking and experience-based design

Patient experience and staff satisfaction have been intrinsically linked with waiting times in the ED (Mortimore and Cooper, 2007). Experience-based design, however, goes beyond canvassing just viewpoints of processes such as wait times. Instead, patients and staff are encouraged to tell their stories of an attendance, and convey emotions and subjective feelings at crucial points along their 'journey'. From these powerful insights opportunities for improvement can be identified and, by working together, patients and staff can redesign these experiences. With lean thinking, individual steps within processes are mapped and areas of waste are identified. Again, this is achieved through the telling of stories of experiences, and then the systematic observation of processes within the department. Combining the two approaches can be a very powerful way to encourage the emergence of innovative improvement solutions.

As healthcare gets to grips with the 21st century, the days of 'doctor always knows best' are over. Our patients are often well informed with access to vast amounts of information about their conditions. The previously paternalistic role of doctors is changing to one of facilitator, helping patients by working with them and providing them with the knowledge they need to make informed collaborative choices. As good clinical leaders, this partnership should not only stop at the consultation, but also focus on the whole patient experience. An important role of clinicians is to co-design and develop services alongside our patients.

Case study

Mike is a Foundation Year Two (F2) doctor working in a busy city centre teaching hospital. In his first few weeks of the job he is often assigned to the minor injury unit. When the department is stretched, other doctors and nurses are often pulled back to the majors area and he is left with a long and growing list of disgruntled patients with minor injuries. He realises that leaving minors to collect equipment needed to suture some of his patients was adding to his time pressure, and that without nursing assistance, this took him considerable time to organise. One busy Thursday night a young man with a facial laceration commented to Mike that it seemed ridiculous he had to keep going forwards and backwards to gather equipment, and that he did not have a pre-designed room with everything he needed to hand.

He discussed this with the emergency nurse practitioner working with him, and as the department quietened down they looked at the setup of the department. They soon noticed design flaws in equipment storage and its accessibility and so thought about ways to improve it. They presented this at a departmental meeting later that week and others added to the discussion with similar frustrated stories. The clinical lead had recently been at a conference and heard how another ED had redesigned the department with lean thinking. A process-mapping workshop was setup and the layout of the department was redesigned. Waiting times dropped significantly and Mike was pleased to report a patient experience survey had already demonstrated more patient satisfaction. On moving to a new Trust, as part his training rotation, he shared this experience of process-mapping and lean thinking.

Setting Direction in the Emergency Department

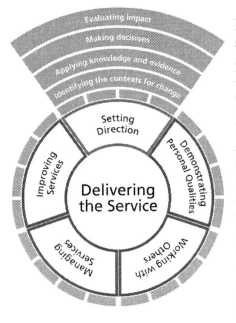

Emergency Medicine as a specialty is relatively young. Accident & Emergency Medicine was first recognised as a specialty in the UK in 1972, and became a College by Royal Charter as recently as 2008 (www.collemergencymed. ac.uk). In thinking about setting the direction of services, the MLCF stipulates that good clinical leaders should apply knowledge and evidence to their practice. Doctors working with the ED will undoubtedly see a vast array of different patients with many different conditions. This variability is what attracts many clinicians to the specialty. However, with such diversity within this thriving but young specialty, it can prove hard for ED doctors to stay on top of recent developments in the conditions they treat. In this section we will look at one way in which the specialty has risen to this challenge, through the formation of an internationally recognised database of best practice in emergency medicine. Much can be learned from the process and indeed the end product.

Applying evidence to improve care

During the 1990s, the ED team at Manchester Royal Infirmary wanted to embed evidence-based practice into the working of the department. They recognised several challenges beyond the wide scope of conditions to be covered. There were no ward rounds, relatively few senior clinicians supervised numerous junior doctors and there was often no senior involvement in individual doctor-patient episodes. Additionally, the department was busy, and taking time to perform a literature search in tackling a clinical conundrum

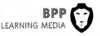

was not feasible on an individual patient basis. Establishing a time-efficient model was key for it to be successful in the ED. It is well worth reading the full story (Carley *et al.*, 1998; Mackway-Jones *et al.*, 1998) but the basics are outlined here.

The team set up a weekly journal club in the department whereby doctors and nurses would meet for one hour with three aims. The first aim was learning how to critically appraise papers. The team ran workshops on how to do this based on *The Pocket Guide to Critical Appraisal* (Crombie, 1996). Armed with these skills, the second aim was to keep on top of current developments in emergency medicine. Given the huge scope covered by the specialty, the choice of journals was honed in to those most relevant and accessible, with certain more relevant and respected journals being reviewed several times in a yearly cycle. Papers within the journals being reviewed were rated by strength of evidence and those rated as the highest quality were presented to the group to influence local practice.

The third aim was to modify an approach whereby a one-page summary of evidence was given to a particular clinical question. With emergency medicine topics often lacking in high quality evidence, they devised a way to formulate the *best available* evidence topic reports. They called these 'BestBETs', aptly reflecting the often uncertain nature of clinical conundrums posed in the ED.

BestBETs

BestBETs are constructed in four stages.

1. First the right **question** is asked and posed in a clinical context. The patient is described, and then an intervention or question is posed to a specified outcome. For example: *in a child with a facial laceration requiring closure, is wound glue better than sutures at improving outcome and reducing the stress of the procedure?*
2. Evidence is **searched** for in readily available electronic databases
3. The evidence is **appraised**
4. Finally, the evidence is **summarised** into a single page

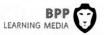

From small beginnings within a department, BestBETs is now an internationally referred-to database. Look it up at www.bestbets.org – it is a great place to start when faced with a clinical conundrum. The scope of BestBETs is now reaching beyond that of emergency medicine and it has helped to develop an international community of clinicians striving to practice in an evidence-based way. If, when you search the database, the answer is not there, get in touch with the team and become an author of a BestBET; it is a great way to contribute and consolidate your understanding and practice of evidence-based medicine (EBM). You could even take it one step further and, by identifying a gap in evidence for a topic, become the pioneer of research into it. Many research projects within the ED have developed in this way.

Embedding evidence-based medicine into clinical work

There are many ways to embed EBM into your work. Regular journal clubs, as demonstrated above, can have far-reaching effects. On a daily basis, challenging yourself and colleagues on why you manage clinical problems in a certain way, and searching BestBETs or other best evidence tools, is a great way to perpetuate your learning, particularly if the condition is unfamiliar to you or if practice has changed. Most EDs will have regular board rounds whereby the team meets at certain times to keep on top of the workload in the department. These meetings are a great opportunity to spend a few minutes updating the team on recent evidence for a topic. If you have been to a course or conference and learned something new, bring it back to the team to share the knowledge and learn together.

Regarding changes in rota patterns (following the introduction of the 48-hour working week for junior doctors) there has been much reported concern about the detrimental effect on training. However, much less is spoken about all of the missed opportunities for experiential learning that occur in every department on a day-to-day basis. The value of learning from informal discussions among colleagues is well recognised (Mayell and Shaw, 2008) and using frameworks such as the BestBET formula can springboard these discussions, as well as leading to the development of a culture where there is a constant search for evidence to improve practice.

Summary

In this chapter we have identified the ED as a busy, stressful and demanding place to work. However, amid the challenges this poses to any doctor in training, there is a myriad of leadership development opportunities available, many of which can happen every day. Debriefing after stressful resuscitations, shadowing the ED registrar, being adaptive to fluctuating workloads and learning alongside others about the best evidence for management of a particular condition are all key examples.

The ED is the gatehouse of the hospital and therefore contains vast numbers of diverse patients. Capitalising on this rich resource and gaining their insight into how services can best be run will bolster innovative solutions to achieving safe, efficient and quality emergency care. The ED has no exclusivity, and sees patients and most clinicians from every specialty group, making many of these learning experiences highly transferable to any part of the healthcare system.

 ### *Three things to try*

1. Think about how you deal with different stressful situations. Are there any other strategies you could develop to support managing stressful situations in the future? Look at the Iverson paper (see references) and see whether any of their suggestions resonate.
2. When you are next involved in a resuscitation or a difficult clinical case, consider whether you are able to initiate or contribute to a team debrief afterwards.
3. Look at the BestBETS website and think about a clinical question which you could write yourself.

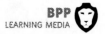

References

Bevan G and Hood C. Have targets improved performance in the English NHS? *BMJ* 2006; 332: 419–422.

Carley SD *et al.* Moving towards evidence based emergency medicine: use of a structures critical appraisal journal club. *J Accid Emerg Med* 1998; 15: 220–226.

The College of Emergency Medicine. Landmarks in the development of the specialty [Online] Available at www.collemergencymed.ac.uk [Accessed 17/10/11].

The College of Emergency Medicine. *CEM welcomes changes to the 4-hour target.* Press Statement – 21st June 2010 [Online] Available at secure.collemergencymed.ac.uk/asp/document.asp?ID=5384 [Accessed 17/10/11].

Crombie IK (1996) *The Pocket Guide to Critical Appraisal.* London: BMJ Publishing Group.

Darzi A (2008) *High Quality Care for All.* NHS Next Stage Review final report [Online] Available at www.dh.gov.uk/en/Publicationsandstatistics/Publications/PublicationsPolicyAndGuidance/DH_085825 [Accessed 17/10/11].

Department of Health (2000) *The NHS Plan, a plan for investment, a plan for reform* [Online] Available at www.dh.gov.uk/en/Publicationsandstatistics/Publications/PublicationsPolicyAndGuidance/DH_4002960 [Accessed 17/10/11].

Department of Health (2001) *NHS performance ratings: Acute Trusts 2000/1* [Online] Available at www.performance.doh.gov.uk/performanceratings/2001/index.html [Accessed 17/10/11].

Department of Health (2010) *Equity and Excellence: Liberating the NHS* [Online] Available at www.dh.gov.uk/en/Publicationsandstatistics/Publications/PublicationsPolicyAndGuidance/DH_117353 [Accessed 17/10/11].

Department of Health (2011) *A&E attendances* [Online] Available at www.dh.gov.uk/en/Publicationsandstatistics/Statistics/Performancedataandstatistics/AccidentandEmergency/DH_077485 [Accessed 17/10/11].

Downing A and Wilson R. Temporal and demographic variations in attendance at accident and emergency departments. *Emerg Med J* 2002; 19: 531–535.

Farhan M. The ABC of handover: a new tool for handover in the emergency department and its impact on practice. *Emerg Med J* 2010; 27: A12.

Fernandez R *et al.* Developing Expert Medical Teams: Toward an Evidence-based Approach. *Academic Emergency Medicine* 2008; 15(11): 1025–1036.

Firth-Cozens J. Doctors, their wellbeing, and their stress. *BMJ (Clinical Research Ed.)* 2003; 326(7391): 670–671.

Firth-Cozens J (1999) The psychological problems of doctors. In Firth-Couzens J and Payne R (eds.) *Stress in health professionals: psychological and organizational causes and interventions.* London: Wiley-Blackwell.

Iversen A, Rushforth B and Forrest K. How to handle stress and look after your mental health. *BMJ* 2009; 338(Apr): b1368–b1368.

Jones JW *et al.* Stress and medical malpractice: organizational risk assessment and intervention. *The Journal of Applied Psychology* 1988; 73(4): 727–735.

Kuhn G, Goldberg R and Compton S. Tolerance for uncertainty, burnout, and satisfaction with the career of emergency medicine. *Annals of Emergency Medicine* 2009; 54(1): 106–113.

Lazarus RS and Folkman S (1984) *Stress, appraisal, and coping.* New York, US: Springer Publishing Company.

Lerner S, Magrane D and Friedman E. Teaching teamwork in medical education. *The Mount Sinai Journal of Medicine, New York* 2009; 76(4): 318–329.

Lowthian J, Curtis A, Cameron P *et al.* Systematic review of trends in emergency department attendances: an Australian perspective. *Emerg Med J* [Online] Available at http://emj.bmj.com/content/early/2010/10/20/emj.2010.099226 [Accessed 17/10/11].

Mackway Jones K, Carley SD, Morton RJ and Donnan S. The best evidence topic report: a modified CAT for summarising the available evidence in emergency medicine. *J Accid Emerg Med* 1998; 15: 222–226.

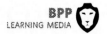

Mayell S and Shaw NJ. Assessing Senior House Officers' Perceptions of Learning. *Arch Dis Child* 2008; 93: 1022–1026.

McCray, LW *et al.* Resident physician burnout: is there hope? *Family Medicine* 2008; 40(9): 626–632.

Mortimore A and Cooper S. The "4-hour target": emergency nurses' views. *Emerg Med J* 2007; 24: 402–404

NHS Institute for Innovation and Improvement. *Experience Based Design* [Online] Available at www.institute.nhs.uk/quality_and_value/introduction/experience_based_design.html [Accessed 17/10/11].

NHS Institute for Innovation and Improvement. *Lean Thinking* [Online] Available at www.institute.nhs.uk/quality_and_value/lean_thinking/lean_thinking.html [Accessed 17/10/11].

Plamping D, Gordon P and Pratt J (2009) *Innovation and Public Services: Insights from Evolution, Whole Systems Working Papers.* Centre for Innovation in Health Management (CIHM) [Online] Available at www.cihm.leeds.ac.uk/new/wp-content/uploads/2009/10/6227_CIHM_public_services_brochure_WEB2.pdf [Accessed 17/10/11].

Rawlinson N. Harms of target driven care. *BMJ* 2008; 337: a885.

Salas E *et al.* Debriefing medical teams: 12 evidence-based best practices and tips. *Joint Commission Journal on Quality and Patient Safety/Joint Commission Resources* 2008; 34(9): 518–527.

Wall T *et al.* Minor psychiatric disorder in NHS trust staff: occupational and gender differences. *The British Journal of Psychiatry* 1997; 171(6): 519–523.

Walley P. Designing the accident and emergency system: lessons from manufacturing. *Emerg Med J* 2003; 20: 126–130.

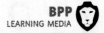

Chapter 8

Leadership Learning In Theatre

Amna Suliman, Bob Klaber
& Oliver Warren

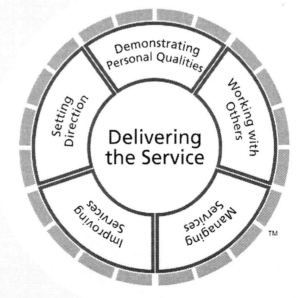

Chapter 8

Leadership Learning in the Operating Theatre

 Chapter overview

This chapter examines the opportunities for leadership learning in theatre, and explores a number of key concepts including:

- Improving patient safety and quality of care
- Developing theatres as a supportive work environment
- Using resources more efficiently
- Using simple low-cost initiatives to improve care
- The importance of values in healthcare
- The processes involved in establishing a 'case for change'

 This chapter also looks at practical tools and techniques which can be used to support learning. These include:

- Leadership measurement tools
- World Health Organization (WHO) safety checklist
- Using audit to drive improvements to care

Introduction

Traditionally, technical ability has been regarded as the single most important skill in the operating theatre, with other attributes such as communication skills and leadership ability deemed significantly less important if not irrelevant. However, the increasing realisation that team interactions and the environment within the operating theatre have demonstrable effects on patient safety and outcomes means that the focus has shifted; the importance of effective leadership in this environment, whether from surgeons, anaesthetists, nurses or other staff continues to be highlighted and clinical practice has started to change. This has provided new opportunities for research, education and development of leadership behaviours and skills.

This chapter uses the five domains of the MLCF to examine what leadership means in the operating theatre and explores the skills and behaviours required to lead effectively in this context. We will explain why these skills are so important, demonstrate how

BPP
LEARNING MEDIA

the operating theatre provides an excellent environment in which to develop them and how this can begin at early career stage. Furthermore, we will illustrate the practical applications of these skills, whether leading the team through a crisis situation during surgery, or more broadly when improving and redesigning services in and around the operating theatre.

Developing leadership skills in the operating theatre

Surgery is a rapidly evolving speciality with constant innovation in surgical techniques, technologies and approaches to delivering care. The operating theatre has changed significantly over time and this changeable environment presents specific challenges to those who lead within it, requiring them to be flexible, open-minded and progressive. We should not expect doctors to have innate leadership skills, at either consultant or trainee level, but these can be successfully developed through persistent input from an early stage in their careers. Opportunities to develop leadership skills should neither be limited to a chosen few nor restricted to people in certain hierarchical roles; instead, as with the model of 'shared leadership' put forward by the MLCF, we should promote leadership within all professionals present in the operating theatre.

The case for developing leadership skills in and around the operating theatre can be based on the following four factors:

1. **Patient safety and quality of care:** wherever improvements or innovations are found in healthcare, it is on the foundation of good clinical leadership. Equally when patients are harmed, as exposed by the inquiries into paediatric cardiac surgery at Bristol Royal Infirmary (The Bristol Royal Infirmary Inquiry, 2001) or patient care at the Mid-Staffordshire Hospital Foundation Trust (Robert Francis Mid-Staffordshire Inquiry, 2010), an absence of clinical leadership is frequently cited as a key contributor. Patient safety is therefore a key reason for leadership to be valued within the operating theatre. Around one in ten patients experience an adverse event during their stay in hospital (Vincent *et al.*, 2001) and in surgery, these mistakes, such as in 'wrong site' surgery, can be catastrophic and cause irreversible harm (Paterson-Brown,

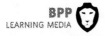

2011). Information transfer in the operating room fails in as many as 30% of communication exchanges (Lingard *et al.*, 2006). Examples such as laryngectomies and mastectomies carried out on the wrong patients have highlighted the need for improving not only leadership but also a range of non-technical skills, such as good communication and ability to work with others, in all staff. Simulations have demonstrated that stress levels fall when communication and leadership is good, resulting in significantly fewer errors and better performance by the operating surgeon. Creating a cohesive theatre team through good leadership may improve outcomes (Hull *et al.*, 2011) and it has been shown that investing in leadership development positively correlates with patient safety and outcomes (Catchpole *et al.*, 2008).

2.   **A supportive work environment:** effective leaders can inspire and enthuse others, and leadership in the operating theatre is no exception to this. Creating a positive 'emotional climate' in theatre can be beneficial to patients and staff (Nurok *et al.*, 2011). Furthermore, negative experiences in theatre, perhaps where there is a serious error or discordance between team members, can take a psychological toll on all involved. A recent study of American surgeons showed one in sixteen had suicidal ideation, the main cause of which was emotional exhaustion (Shanafelt, 2011). Anecdotal evidence suggests surgeons suffer psychological harm if they are involved in inadvertently harming patients or failures of care.

3.   **More efficient use of resources:** as highlighted in the *Managing Services* domain of the MLCF, successfully managing resources (both human and economic) are important leadership competencies. The worsening financial constraints on healthcare, caused by both economic downturn and healthcare inflation being persistently higher than standard inflation, have created an increasing need for doctors to feel as comfortable with financial accountability as they do with clinical decisions. In the operating theatre poor leadership may result in overbooking the operating lists, late finishing and paying staff overtime to stay late. Likewise under-utilisation may also occur, wasting resources and opportunity. Although many surgeons feel uncomfortable with the idea

of considering costs when operating, they are responsible for spending significant sums of money, particularly if choosing grafts, prosthesis or certain equipment. By choosing the most expensive option, which may have no measurable benefit to the individual, a surgeon may inadvertently impact on the availability of resources to a wider population of patients (Stanton *et al.*, 2011). Learning how to make these decisions and to articulate them to others within the team is an important part of leadership within the operating theatre.

4. **Shaping the local environment and influencing healthcare decisions:** medical practitioners at all levels of seniority should contribute to improvements in the quality of service within their speciality; this undoubtedly includes surgeons and anaesthetists within the operating theatre (Warren and Carnall, 2011). In some areas of healthcare within the UK there seems to be an increasing desire from junior doctors and consultants to improve their working environment, alongside an increasing belief that health services do better when doctors become involved in leading healthcare services or organisations (Stoll *et al.*, 2010). Elsewhere in the world, doctor-led organisations are considered more routine, with around 30% of healthcare chief executives also being doctors in the USA, compared to less than 5% in the NHS (Griffiths, 1983). Political reform continues to mirror this movement towards clinician leadership with politicians describing a desire to shift accountability for the commissioning of services, and design of patients' care pathways, away from managers towards doctors. These changes, along with a potentially liberated marketplace, may result in surgeons, anaesthetists and operating department staff working for different organisations in the future, or establishing and leading their own chambers or provider organisations (Garside and Black, 2003). It is suggested that most surgeons are currently ill-equipped to do this and those with the best leadership and managerial skills, and experience, are the people most likely to get the best for their patients in such an environment.

The operating theatre as a learning environment

As explained earlier, leadership has undergone a series of definitions and re-definitions with time in an attempt to harness its real meaning in the context of healthcare. Figure 8.1 illustrates one of the many classifications of leadership theories, though there are many others that have been described. Everyone knows equally effective leaders who have entirely contrasting styles; this makes it difficult to create a uniform prototype or role model. Leadership is a multifaceted and pliable concept, adaptable to the individual, organisation and environment in which it occurs (in this case, the operating theatre).

Leadership measurement tools

As the importance of leadership has grown in recognition, numerous measurement tools have been developed or adapted from other industries to assess leadership in the operating theatre, usually as one of many 'non-technical skills'. The most widely used of these assessment systems include:

- The Non-Technical Skills for Surgeons (NOTSS) scale is an observational behaviour-rating tool looking at surgeons during an operation (Yule *et al.*, 2006). This analyses leadership specifically as one of its four categories alongside the surgeon's ability to 'cope with pressure', 'support others' and 'set/ maintain standards'.
- The Non-Technical Skills for Pilots (NOTECHS) scale (Sevdalis *et al.*, 2008; Flin *et al.*, 2003) is adapted from the aviation industry and defines leadership as adherence to best practice during the procedure, time management, resource utilisation, debriefing, authority and assertiveness. A revised NOTECHS scale has also been implemented in surgery for use in crisis simulation (Undre *et al.*, 2007).
- Observational Teamwork Assessment for Surgery (OTAS) is an observational tool looking at the multidisciplinary contributions within the operating theatre (Healey *et al.*, 2004). It defines leadership as 'provision of direction, assertiveness and support of team members.'

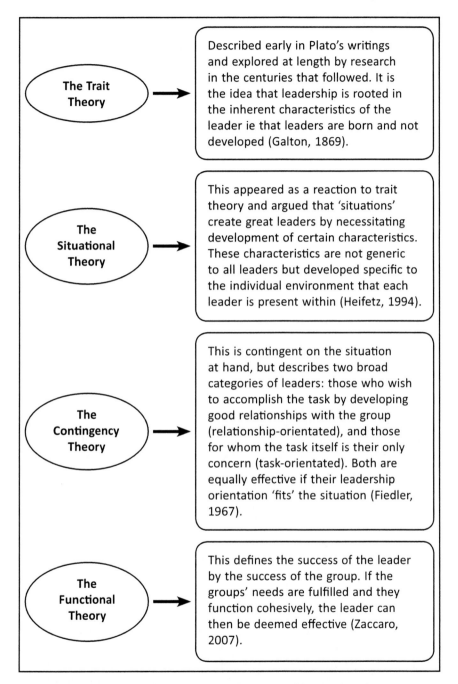

Figure 8.1 One of the many classifications of leadership theories

There is significant overlap in the qualities these tools highlight as important in the operating theatre with those generically outlined in the Medical Leadership Competency Framework (MLCF). However, tools such as NOTSS, NOTECHS and OTAS broadly address 'non-technical skills', a term meant to encompass all attributes apart from what the surgeons' hands are doing. There are very few studies looking exclusively at leadership in the operating theatre. Not only this, but several simulation studies have recognised that these skills often degenerate and cannot withstand stressful intra-operative scenarios in theatre (Wetzel *et al.*, 2010), paradoxically the worst time for them to diminish. Most commonly, the operating surgeon is leading the team, dictating the aims, direction and pace of the procedure while at the same time, along with the anaesthetist, being the individual most aware of the patient's condition and needs. However, in specific situations leadership may need to be transferred seamlessly between team members ie the anaesthetist-surgeon-perfusionist-nurse. This makes inclusion of leadership capability, as part of the assessment and continuing professional development of surgeons, anaesthetists and senior theatre nurses, of vital importance.

The 'micro-environment' of theatre

When considering ideas about leadership learning in theatre, you should consider the MLCF domains within the context of the operating theatre and appreciate the uniqueness of this environment. It is a relatively small, enclosed space which creates an intense 'micro-environment', often hotter, more humid and noisier than a normal office space, clinic or ward. Events within it can be greatly unpredictable, with regular changes of pace, people and concentration levels. Stress levels in individuals and within the team itself can fluctuate rapidly. Subsequent interactions between the team can potentially become chaotic and unclear, leading to crises. Managing this safely and efficiently requires impeccable communication, teamwork and leadership, and it is within this context that the opportunities for leadership learning within theatre should be examined. Figure 8.2 outlines some of the key qualities outlined by the MLCF that are perhaps most relevant specifically to the operating theatre, and looks at examples of how they can be developed to achieve more effective leadership in this area.

Key for Figure 8.2

SS	=	Senior Surgeon (Consultant/Registrar)
JrS	=	Surgical SHO/HO/Student
SA	=	Senior Anaesthetist (Consultant/Registrar)
JrAn	=	Anaesthetics SHO/HO/Student
ODP	=	Operating Departmental Practitioners
SN	=	Scrub Nurse, Nursing Assistants
TN	=	Theatre Nurses
WS	=	Ward Staff
P	=	Patient
TM	=	Theatre Manager
Rel	=	Patient relatives
DH	=	Department of Health

MLCF Competency and Domain	Potential leaders/Team members	Behaviours/Skills	Examples in the Operating Theatre
Ensuring patient safety ('Improving Services')	SS JrS SA JrA TN SN ODP WS P	Meticulousness Attention to detail Patient-centeredness Communication Education Governance and use of guidelines Technical competence	Use of WHO patient safety checklist Thrombo-prophylaxis administration Antibiotic prescription at induction Clear Consenting and marking Appropriate choice of operation Appropriate type of anaesthetic Safe transfer Clear operation note and post-operative instructions
Encouraging improvement and innovation ('Improving Services')	SS JrS SA JrA TN SN WS TM DH	Familiarity with guidelines Audit and Governance Education of juniors in the importance of patient experience and patient journey Flexibility Patient-centeredness Progressiveness Evidence based practise	Keeping up to date with literature/techniques/courses Educational/blame free culture in Morbidity and Mortality meetings Encouraging junior involvement in audit and analysis of intra-operative events/outcomes Promote involvement in managerial role in hospital/Trust/DH from young stage
Working with teams ('Working with Others')	SA JrA SS JrS	Support and value others and their contributions Flexibility/adaptability Listening and communication	Courtesy when giving instructions/making requests (surgeon/scrub nurse/anaesthetist) Communication and agreement when team is 'ready to send for next patient' or 'ready to start

Figure 8.2 Key MLCF qualities and examples of how they can be developed

MLCF Competency and Domain	Potential leaders/Team members	Behaviours/Skills	Examples in the Operating Theatre
Working with teams ('Working with Others') continued	SN TN ODP WS TM P Rel	Encouraging and nurturing individual specialist interests Delegation Clear communication Leading by example Teaching and training Approachability and availability	operation' Helping transfer patient and set up theatre Calm cohesive teamwork in a crisis Introductions/debriefing/regular forum for discussion of how team can evolve and improve.
Building and maintaining relationships ('Working with Others')	SS SA JrS JrA SN ODP TM P Rel WS	Patience Sincerity/kindness Team worker Supportive in a crisis Constructive feedback Clear and polite communication	Well planned lists that do not overrun/considerate of other staff members Patient-centeredness and teamwork when delays/complications arise Encouraging and approachable to students/juniors Not hurrying surgeon in view of sending for next patient Surgeons having patience when equipment malfunctions or long induction Carrying out assessments for juniors
Encouraging contribution ('Working with Others')	SS SA JrS JrA SN	Approachability Availability Constructive feedback and re-assessment Patience	Allow junior/student to suture/intubate Allow Registrar to attempt complex anastomosis Gentle questioning and teaching Team discussion about order of list/type of anaesthetic/best use of theatre time

Figure 8.2 Key MLCF qualities and examples of how they can be developed

MLCF Competency and Domain	Potential leaders/Team members	Behaviours/Skills	Examples in the Operating Theatre
Encouraging contribution ('Working with Others') continued	TM DH	Listening and communication skills Adaptability	Set targets and check goals are achieved as a team Welcome variation/alternative approaches/techniques
Developing self-awareness ('Developing Personal Qualities')	SS SA JrS JrA SN ODP TM	Recognising own strengths/weaknesses/limits Knowing own role and that of others Emotional intelligence Communication and listening Flexibility/adaptability with situation Knowing when to lead/step back	Fulfilling role as lead surgeon/assistant effectively Supporting junior members and being aware of what else is going on in the room (anaesthetic changes/instructions) Identifying teaching opportunities Knowing when to give opinion/feedback and when not to Clear instructions to others Familiarity with equipment and flexibility with shortages Ability to handle challenges/crisis and knowing when to ask for help
Managing performance ('Managing Services')	SS SA Jr A JrS SN TM DH	Valuing and encouraging new ideas Setting clear goals and expectations Regular assessment/audit of practise. Giving constructive feedback Clear communication and listening	Incident reporting Carrying out work-based assessments Team meetings/debriefings Giving clear instructions Pre-ordering and checking equipment WHO check list

Figure 8.2 Key MLCF qualities and examples of how they can be developed

MLCF Competency and Domain	Potential leaders/Team members	Behaviours/Skills	Examples in the Operating Theatre
Managing resources (Managing Services')	SS SA JrS JrA SN ODP TM P Rel WS	Business acumen Prioritisation Clinical knowledge Flexibility Sensitive to needs of others and advice of team Patient centred approach Evidence-based practise	Requesting correct equipment and checking to prevent opening new sets Prudent use of ITU/HDU Employment of theatre staff and hours Bed management/day surgery
Managing people (Managing Services')	SS SA TM SN DH	Fluent communication and clear instructions Valuing opinions of others Adaptable Approachable Delegation Knowledgeable Able to lead by example Educates and explains reasons behind decisions/actions/urgency	Explain how and why list is a specific order Decide on equipment needs early and be organised Constructive feedback regarding errors/incidents Be an advocate for patient safety and patient experience Teach and support juniors (give individual's specific roles according to their knowledge base/interest)

Figure 8.2 Key MLCF qualities and examples of how they can be developed

Demonstrating Personal Qualities in the operating theatre

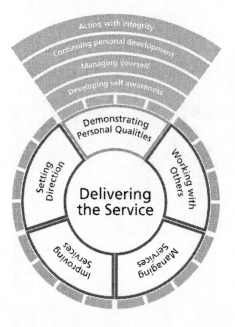

The operating theatre team are the ultimate example of a group of individuals who, no matter how good their individual competencies, cannot succeed without their colleagues. The ability to work together and trust in one another is essential. A surgeon can rarely operate without an anaesthetist, a scrub nurse or an assistant, and so any person unable to work with others, to lead others and to engender loyalty and respect will find themselves significantly impaired in this environment. Fundamental to achieving this trust, respect and teamworking are strong personal qualities as highlighted in the *Demonstrating Personal Qualities* domain of the MLCF. This entails self-awareness, managing oneself, supporting learning and professional development, and behaving in an open, honest and ethical manner.

 Exercise 8.1   **Scenario**

Adela is a very experienced matron who has been the scrub nurse for Professor Chan's elective orthopaedic list for many years. She is extremely familiar and comfortable with even his most complex procedures. Recently Adela has been asked to train one of the more junior nurses in scrubbing in with total hip replacements; however she is nervous about broaching this subject with Professor Chan. He becomes visibly uncomfortable when assisted by anyone else and is not particularly patient if there are pauses or omissions. She feels torn between her duties as a trainer and her reluctance to disrupt the list by allowing a less experienced nurse to scrub in. She wishes communication was more open and that he was more approachable and respectful of her desire to develop other members of the team.

Image © 2010 NHS Institute and AoMRC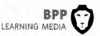

Exercise 8.1 *(Continued)*   **Scenario**

- How might Adela approach this issue?
- How can training occur without unduly affecting team performance under time pressure?

Summary of issues

This scenario, where the prospect of any change causes alarm and discontent for a team that works successfully together, is not an unusual one. A change in colleagues who you trust, respect and have learned to rely on, such as a certain theatre sister or anaesthetist, can often lead to anxiety which may make the environment uncomfortable if expressed. In this example, if Professor Chan wants to have a team that is sustainable and not overly reliant on any given individual, he will need to find a way to support the training of a new theatre nurse. Additionally, Adela needs to empathise and acknowledge his eagerness to get through a whole list on time, and not unnecessarily lengthen any patient's operation. A compromise might be to allow the trainee to initially do one case a day.

The importance of values

Similar scenarios arise in all departments, with surgical core trainees eager to suture wounds or anaesthetic trainees eager to intubate. A key part of working successfully with others is being able to acknowledge and respect their needs and values, empathise with them and be kind and patient. Communication and self-awareness are key to achieving this. It is also important to be clear, from the very beginning of any working relationship, that supporting personal development and developing new members of a team are core values. Seeking regular feedback from experienced and junior team members about how everyone feels, promoting open discussion and preventing any silent build-up of resentment are also vital steps in protecting team morale.

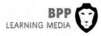

Working with Others in the operating theatre

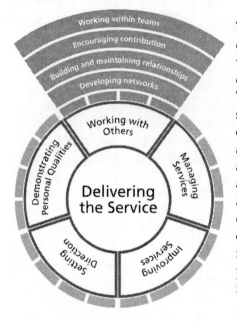

The MLCF describes how doctors show leadership by working within teams to deliver and improve services. This means each individual should have a clear sense of their role, responsibilities and purpose within the team, and adopt a supportive team approach which acknowledges and appreciates the efforts, contributions and compromises of others. Fundamental to this is recognising the common purpose of the team and respecting team decisions.

 Exercise 8.2   **Scenario**

Sally is a Foundation Year 1 (F1) doctor who begins her first four-month rotation as a doctor in cardiothoracic surgery under Mr Wilson. She attends the full day list of thoracic cases each Friday and always gets the feeling that the mood in theatre is tense or uncomfortable, and morale is low. She begins to reflect on what contributes to this and picks out a number of individual frustrations and character traits leading to the negative atmosphere. The nurses feel Mr Wilson's list always overruns significantly so that Friday evenings are often spent in the hospital instead of at home with their families. Mr Wilson is frustrated as he feels Dr Levi, the anaesthetist, takes too long putting patients to sleep in between cases, and since there are four cases, this prolongs the list. Dr Levi feels dejected by how, despite repeatedly asking to send for the next patient, there is often a delay as nurses are preoccupied, porters unavailable and on arrival the patients often are often inadequately prepared.

> **Exercise 8.2** *(Continued)* **Scenario**
> - How can developing a strong approach to working with others improve the situation in this operating theatre?
> - What role can Sally take to maintain changes to a healthier emotional climate in theatre?

Summary of issues

This common scenario is an example of how each individual's personal characteristics and expectations of others can limit the functionality of the team and hamper productivity. In a scenario where there is widespread dissatisfaction, a group forum, where all opinions can be heard, can significantly help.

World Health Organization (WHO) safety checklist

The recently introduced World Health Organization (WHO) safety checklist recommends introductions before, and debriefing after, each case. This may address some of the issues here. If the new and existing team members introduced themselves each Friday morning, this would start some early interactions. Stating individual requests and group strategies for the day such as 'aiming to send promptly for each patient', 'finish at a sensible time' or 'allowing each person adequate breaks' provides a clear plan for all. It is also an opportunity to outline the correct equipment needed for each case, and any other issues that may impact on the planned work. In debriefing sessions, any concerns or frustrations can be constructively voiced and positive group or individual behaviours can be acknowledged.

Using audit to stimulate change

While initiating this would be a significant challenge for a very junior doctor, inexperience and *perceived naivety* is sometimes beneficial, allowing gentle questioning of someone's understanding of practice. There is also great scope for the most junior team member to energise those around them with their fresh perspective, energy and commitment to developing as a doctor. In this example, to add to her credibility, Sally could initiate a formal audit of how frequently the list finishes late and identify where the delays lie. She could then work with colleagues to make specific suggestions, such as allocating one person to send for patients at the correct time, or ensuring ward teams fully prepare patients pre-operatively or that they are given an early warning call. The audit could be repeated by the next FY1 doctor in the months after the implementation of these changes. Through these strategies, positive interactions and contributions can be encouraged and the team can hopefully deliver safer, more efficient care within a stress-free environment.

Managing Services in the operating theatre

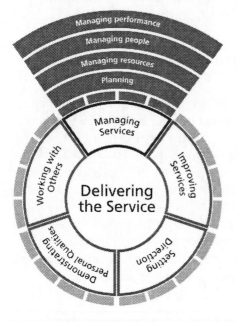

All clinicians working in theatres, whether surgeons, anaesthetists, nurses or ODPs, are somewhat involved in managing the services they provide. The MLCF describes planning *services* and managing *people*, *performance* and *resources* as the four key elements of this domain. The following example of service management explores the role of a clinician in managing resources and improving efficiency.

Exercise 8.3 — Scenario

Miss Castle is a consultant breast surgeon who has been newly appointed to a department with financial difficulties. During her first few weeks she tries to ascertain how her department procures implants for reconstruction following mastectomies. To her surprise, she finds many different types of implant are being ordered, due to the individual preference of each consultant. They are often therefore ordered individually, or in low volume, thus preventing any significant cost reductions from the suppliers. She calculates the amount that could be saved if everyone conformed to just two types, and discovers that this would save the Trust thousands of pounds each year. She then starts to think how she could gain her colleagues' support for this change.

- How could Miss Castle effect this change within her department?
- How can junior team members become involved in managing theatre services?

Summary of issues

Miss Castle first needs to ensure her information is accurate by enlisting the help of her theatre manager colleagues and the prosthesis company representatives, and perhaps consider getting a colleague or friend to check her figures. She needs to be able to connect this financial information to any clinical outcome data or patient experience feedback that may also impact on the decision-making. Rather than trying to change things informally, she may achieve more by presenting her case at a divisional or departmental meeting, maybe having already recruited a like-minded colleague to encourage or support her. She needs to think ahead and predict who might be resistant to this change and consider why, allowing her to prepare counter-arguments. Demonstrating empathy and understanding the perspective of others, while having a clear understanding of the clinical and financial arguments, would allow her to be effective in any negotiation. She needs to be open that there is no personal gain for her in this change, but that the department may be more secure as a result of the financial savings. Additionally, actively welcoming ideas from her colleagues (both clinical and managerial) about where else the money may then be used would be another way of gaining support.

Getting involved with service management

Service management need not be restricted to consultants. Staff and Associate Specialist grade doctors and trainees should be encouraged to think they have a role too. Audits, seen as essential for building a strong personal learning portfolio, can be focused on the way the service treats its patients. Examples of this might be auditing re-attendance after day surgery, or the time from booking emergency cases to them actually occurring. This may lead to suggestions for improvement. Other trainees may want to focus on using their 'on the ground' knowledge and insights to support their management colleagues in streamlining services and exploring other potential efficiency gains. Commissioning and developing training programmes where the responsibility for contributing to, and learning about, the management of a service is an inherent component of all doctors' roles and is likely to promote more proactive, financially sound and clinically engaged departments in the future.

Improving Services in the operating theatre

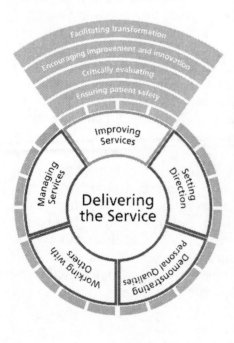

Improving services in the operating theatre can be as simple as concentrating on transferring patients safely, positioning them in a way that will not expose them to injury or cold, or improving theatre utilisation by ensuring patients are moved from the recovery area to the wards as soon as clinically appropriate. It can however include much larger change programmes, such as the acquisition of new, sophisticated machinery, instruments and camera equipment or installing state of the art elective orthopaedic surgery suites. The following example demonstrates how a small improvement in a service can have a cascade effect on improving the patient experience and outcome.

Exercise 8.4   Scenario

A patient, Mrs Tadros, is admitted from A&E for a laparoscopic appendicectomy. In theatre the procedure is undertaken by the on-call surgical registrar and goes smoothly. However, the surgeon's bleep goes off throughout the procedure with urgent requests for opinions throughout the hospital. Upon finishing the operation she therefore hurries her operation note and departs to see the patients waiting elsewhere. When Mrs Tadros is transferred to the ward, the nurses are unable to read the surgeon's writing and cannot make out the post-operative instructions, which means Mrs Tadros does not receive the desired antibiotics. The next day, the emergency team are unsure of any further instructions, reluctant to discharge her too early and uncertain whether she should have any antibiotics. The junior doctor doing the discharge summary is unclear about whether any follow-up is required. To avoid missing anything, he books an outpatient appointment.

- What are the potential consequences of illegible operation notes?
- What steps might be taken to prevent these problems?
- Can you think of any other examples where small changes to theatre processes may improve outcomes for patients?

Summary of issues

As this example demonstrates, illegible operation notes may result in harm to patients. While in this case the actual harm done was minor, it was significant enough to involve missing medication and possibly a lengthened hospital stay, both of which have increased Mrs Tadros' chance of infective morbidity following this procedure. She will also attend an unnecessary follow-up appointment. This illustrates that small deficits in one element of theatre performance can have significant consequences for patients and cost the provider financially.

Improving care through simple low-cost initiatives

To address this, leaders in the operating theatre may try to standardise processes (eg designated operating theatres for designated specialities; tick-box options on operation notes), create default positions (eg all vascular patients receive anti-coagulation therapy unless the consultant states otherwise; no case cancelled without clinical director involvement), and make small design changes to facilitate communication (eg day surgery unit next door to theatres; portable telephones for key staff members). Relatively minor changes can make large differences in cancellation rates, unnecessary follow-ups and variations in care. For example, as happens in some hospitals, a surgeon could make a brief telephone call to a nominated family member at the end of every major case, to ensure they know what has happened in the operating theatre and to give them immediate feedback about how their relative is. This is a good example of a near-zero cost intervention that can have a significant impact on patient and carer satisfaction. These sorts of improvements should therefore remain a focus for anyone wanting to be an effective leader in the theatre. Whether you are a medical student, trainee, or newly appointed consultant, getting involved with improvement projects like these is undoubtedly the best way to learn about and experience change.

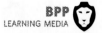

Setting Direction in the operating theatre

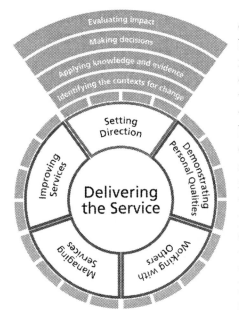

Changes in surgical services, both unscheduled and elective, may occur when new members of staff are appointed. They will bring their own ideas of what methods to use, often based on what they have seen elsewhere. Existing teams should also be encouraged to regularly review and reassess their current practice and performance, and set new goals or take new strategic direction to achieve better results for their patients and ensure the long-term viability of their service.

Exercise 8.5   Scenario

Dr Mohsen is a consultant anaesthetist and clinical director of surgery, anaesthetics and intensive care. He is aware that many of the trust's elective surgical cases are being cancelled or delayed due to an expanding emergency workload, which is only likely to increase because of the closure of the neighbouring ED. Furthermore, the wait for emergency patients to receive their operation appears to be increasing. Dr Mohsen worries about the impact this has on the quality of care the hospital provides, and the financial implications for the Trust.

- How might Dr Mohsen improve the current situation?
- How can he use his colleagues to help him?

Summary of issues

Dr Mohsen needs to create a 'case for change'. It might be that other colleagues may not have fully recognised the issues. If he can convince others within the Trust that there is a problem, he is more likely to create a vision for future theatre services and set a direction for his service. To this end he starts to collect data; his trainees do some of this as they perform audits exploring the 'time to operation' from the booking of emergency cases; his theatre manager collects some too, demonstrating patterns in the cancellations and sharing national targets for elective procedure cancellation rates and their arrangements with local commissioners. Dr Mohsen also consults guidelines on emergency surgery from bodies such as the Royal College of Surgeons, and identifies what other successful organisations are doing in this area by using his professional networks.

Once Dr Mohsen creates a compelling series of arguments as to why something needs to be done (a 'case for change'), he develops some possible solutions. Some are focused on the short-term and are relatively simple, eg changes to National Confidential Enquiry into Patient Outcome and Death (NCEPOD) list timings and the ring-fencing of one ward for purely elective admissions. Others involve how the ideal scenario may look and how the Trust might get there eg a complete elective and emergency split, using their off-site treatment centre and the creation of two new consultant posts in emergency surgery. Finally, he tries to enact his change through others by recruiting colleagues to champion this vision. This requires him to work across professional boundaries by engaging a well-respected bed manager and the lead nurse for theatres, who are both desperate for something to change. Together they present options to the Board and give the staff the belief that there is a long-term vision for the service.

While the leadership of an initiative with such scope will come from a senior leader, there are many opportunities in Exercise 8.5 where trainees and other team members can contribute to the development of the case for change, and the solutions that may follow.

Summary

Operating theatres provide an excellent micro-environment for the study and development of behaviours and non-technical skills. It is a stressful, emotional and rapidly changing environment and therefore one where leadership behaviour plays an important role in effective performance. Strong leaders, equipped with a broad range of skills, not only increase patient safety and theatre efficiency but also promote happier, healthier teams.

Few doctors work solely in an operating department setting, but as we have demonsrated, the operating theatre is an excellent environment to develop leadership skills and experience. Embracing these learning opportunities will not only develop individual capabilities but also ensure a positive environment for all team members involved and, above all, improve outcomes and experience for patients.

 Three things to try

1. Consider how you can use an audit of current practice to build a case for change that will lead to improvements in the quality of care and patient experience.
2. Ask key family members if they would appreciate a brief telephone call from you or a member of the surgical team as soon as their relative's operation is over.
3. The next time you are involved in a team simulation of any kind, ask the facilitators to specifically feedback the effectiveness of your leadership behaviours during it.

References and further reading

Catchpole K, Mishra A and Handa A *et al*. Teamwork and error in the operating room: Analysis of skills and roles. *Ann Surg* 2008; 247: 699–706.

Department of Health. *Robert Francis Inquiry Report into Mid-Staffordshire NHS Foundation Trust* [Online] Available at www.dh.gov.uk/er/Publications and statistics/Publications/PublicationsPolicyAndGuidance/DH_113018 [Accessed 17/10/11].

Fiedler Fred E (1967) *A theory of leadership effectiveness*. McGraw-Hill: Harper and Row Publishers Inc.

Flin R, Martin L and Goeters K *et al*. Development of NOTECHS (non-technical skills) system for rating pilots' CRM skills. *Human Factors and Aerospace Safety* 2003; 3: 95–117.

Galton F (1869) *Hereditary Genius*. London: Macmillan.

Garside P and Black A. Doctors in chambers. *BMJ* 2003; Mar 22; 326(7390): 611–2.

Griffiths R (1983) *NHS Management Enquiry*. London: DHSS; HMSO.

Healey AN, Undre S and Vincent CA. Developing observational measures of performance in surgical teams. *Qual Safe Health Care* 2004; 13 (Suppl 1) i33–40.

Heifetz R (1994) *Leadership without Easy Answers*. Cambridge, MA: Harvard University Press.

Hull L *et al.* Assessment of stress and teamwork in the operating room: an exploratory study. *Am J Surg* 2011; 201: 24–30.

Lingard L, Espin S and Whyte S *et al.* A theory-based instrument to evaluate team communication in the operating room: observational classification of recurrent types and effects. *Qual Saf Health Care* 2006; 15: 422–426.

Nurok M, Evans LA and Lipsitz S *et al.* The relationship of the emotional climate of work and threat to patient outcome in a high-volume thoracic surgery operating room team. *BMJ Qual Saf* [Online] Available at qualitysafety.bmj.com/content/early/2011/01/04/bmjqs.2009.039008 [Accessed 17/10/11].

Patel VM *et al.* What does leadership in surgery entail? *Anz J Surg* 2010; 80(12): 876–83.

Paterson-Brown, S. Improving patient safety through education. *BMJ* 2011; 342: d214.

Sevdalis N, Davis R and Koutantji M *et al.* Reliability of a revised NOTECHS scale for use in surgical teams. *Am J Srg* 2008; 196: 184–90.

Shanafelt TD *et al.* Special report: suicidal ideation among American surgeons. *Arch Surg* 2011; 146: 54–62.

Stanton E, Lemer C and Marshall M. An evolution of professionalism. *J R Soc Med* 2011; 104: 48–9.

Stoll L, Foster-Turner J and Glenn M (2010) *Mind Shift: an evaluation of the NHS London 'Darzi' Fellowships in Clinical Leadership Programme*. London: London Deanery [Online] Available at www.ioe.ac.uk/IOE_Fellowship_evaluation_report_final_July_2010.pdf [Accessed 17/10/11].

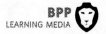

The Bristol Royal Infirmary Inquiry (2001) *Learning from Bristol: the report of the public inquiry into children's heart surgery at the Bristol Royal Infirmary 1984–1995* [Online] Available at www.bristol-inquiry.org.uk [Accessed 17/10/11]

Under S, Koutantji M and Sevdalis N *et al.* Multidisciplinary crisis simulations: The way forward for training surgical teams. *World J Surg* 2007; 31: 1843–5.

Vincent C, Neale G and Woloshynowych M. Adverse events in British hospitals: preliminary retrospective record review. *BMJ* 2001; 322: 517–9.

Warren O and Carnall R. Medical Leadership: why it's so important, what is required and how we develop it. *Postgrad Med J* [Online] Available at http://pmj.bmj.com/content/87/1023/27.full [Accessed 17/10/11].

Wetzel C *et al.* The Effects of Stress and Coping on Surgical Performance during Simulations. *Ann Surg* 2010; 251: 171–176.

World Alliance for Patient Safety (2009) *The WHO Surgical Safety Checklist* [Online] Available at www.who.int/patientsafety/safesurgery/ss_checklist/en/index.html [Accessed 17/10/11].

Yule S, Flin R and Paterson-Brown S *et al.* Development of a rating system for surgeons' non-technical skills. *Med Educ* 2006; 40: 1098–104.

Zaccaro S J. Trait-Based Perspectives of Leadership. *Am Psychol* 2007; 62(1): 6–16.

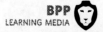

Demonstrating Personal Qualities in Primary Care

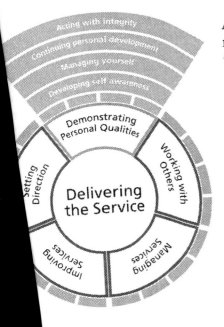

As highlighted in Chapter 7, regarding Emergency Medicine, the stress and pressure felt by doctors and other healthcare workers can be huge. A key element of the *Demonstrating Personal Qualities* domain of the MLCF focuses on managing yourself. This area of leadership has many parallels with clinical practice. There are a lot of support systems in place for clinicians, particularly GPs, who find themselves under stress whether that is work-related, financial or outside of work (British Medical Association, 2011). However, we as individuals know the warning signs, we risk missing ance to avert problems before they escalate.

ging stress

care, like much of medicine, is a stressful place to work: ns are often important and inherently risky, with little if they turn out to be wrong. Clinicians work largely on n with very variable support systems; the working day is sy with little time to discuss problems. Additionally, the ous nature of many clinicians makes them loathe to share over work. Among other issues, doctors are more likely rest of the population to suffer from one or more of 'the drugs, drink and depression (and a higher risk of suicide). tend to try to work through illness, resist seeking help he usual channels and frequently self-prescribe (British ssociation, 2007).

BPP LEARNING MEDIA

Chapter 9

Leadership Learning in Primary Care

David Griffiths

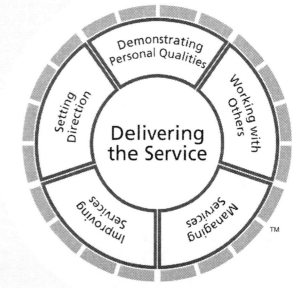

Leadership Learning in Primary Care

Chapter overview

This chapter examines the opportunities for leadership learning in general practice, and explores a number of key concepts including:

- The traditional model of the 1:1 consultation
- Developing networks
- Building and managing relationships
- Developing planning skills
- Involving colleagues to accomplish change
- Clinical engagement and the dangers of disengagement
- Evidence-based service improvement

This chapter also looks at practical tools and techniques which can be used to support learning. These include:

- Safety-netting and housekeeping checkpoints
- Networking
- Mindmaps
- Stakeholder mapping
- PDSA cycles
- Process mapping and value stream mapping
- The clinical engagement ladder

Introduction

There are approximately 41,000 GPs in the UK, delivering around 250 million consultations per year. The GP workforce is extremely varied, including partners, salaried and sessional GPs, retainers, returners, GPs with specialist interests (GPSIs), Primary Care Trusts (PCT) and Strategic Health Authority (SHA) clinical advisors, medicolegal experts, and many more. With the rise of portfolio careers (where GPs take on two or more roles simultaneously), and an increasingly part-time workforce, the need for leaders in general practice and primary care is greater than ever.

There is already a cadre of experienced and effective GP leaders, but there is also an argument that their generation is out of touch with the next, which could have serious implications for the future.

The traditional model of leadership training, the GP has become less common since the introduction of contract which encouraged partners to take on sala

General practice now and in the future

The 'model' of UK general practice – 1:1 consul doctor – has changed little over the last 30 years some practices now use, for example, telephone t nurse practitioners, email, or text alerts, many oth predominantly working in a traditional flat struct to change significantly over the next 10 years.

General practice is often referred to as a mult setting and yet most of the multidisciplinary separately in 'silos', discussing cases only rare particular need (eg the signing of a prescription of a dressing). This does not make the most o available and needs to change.

> *The basic unit of activity will no lon consultation with a doctor but the provisio multidisciplinary service that pro-active managing their own health.*

(*Improving the Quality of*

There is considerable resistance to change based on a belief that the consultation is places, due to lack of trust and confidenc in quality improvement other than audit model of 1:1 consultations leaves little t particularly for less than full-time wor for general practice: how can we give t GPs the opportunity to lead; to push i (eg integrating with secondary car patient-centred; and to inspire and GP leaders?

unless
the ch

Man

Primar
decisio
backup
their ow
often b
autonon
or hand
than the
three Ds'
They als
through
Medical

In leadership roles, these issues are just as pressing and decisions may be even more important. Leaders often remain, to some extent, apart from their team in order to keep clear boundaries. Balancing clinical and managerial commitments can be extremely challenging and, particularly in times of financial austerity, there may be no-one to share work and responsibility with.

To use a parallel with clinical practice, it is worth looking to one of the most respected GPs in the UK, Roger Neighbour, a former chair of the RCGP. His book, *The Inner Consultation* (Neighbour, 2005), is possibly the highest profile book on 'the consultation'. Neighbour's consultation model consists of five 'checkpoints', two of which are particularly relevant to the idea of managing oneself.

Neighbour's checkpoints: safety-netting

The first checkpoint to consider is *safety-netting*. The intention is to reduce the risk of adverse events if any decision turns out to be wrong. GPs should qualify their management plan by asking themselves three questions:

1. What do I expect to happen?
2. What will happen if I'm wrong?
3. What would I do then?

These three questions then form the basis for a safe management plan for the patient, and the communication of the safety net is a key part of many GPs' consultation style. In the era of patient-centred practice, this is an important way to empower patients.
If we extend this practice to leadership, there are similar potential benefits. Developing a clear strategy, with equally clear contingency arrangements for where things do not go exactly according to plan, both reduces the stress for ourselves as leaders and empower our teams to carry on and work independently.

Neighbour's checkpoints: housekeeping

A second, and perhaps even more important checkpoint, is that of *housekeeping*. Neighbour reminds us that, as humans, GPs (and indeed all clinicians) are susceptible to stress, tiredness, boredom, hunger, irritation and many other emotions. It is part of our professional responsibility as clinicians to make sure we are in the best possible state for every patient we see, and we should not consider a consultation 'over' until we are ready for the next one. This may not be relevant after every consultation but it is important to recognise when it *is* an issue.

Leaders are, of course, prone to emotions too. As with *safety-netting*, the concept of *housekeeping* is a useful one for the aspiring leader. Any role involving logical thought and clear decision-making obviously requires a clear head. What is more, as previously stated, leadership roles are inherently stressful and can frequently push someone into uncomfortable situations. There is no question that the best leaders will have ways of dealing with stress in order to function at their best, whether they are explicit about them or not.

Case study

Dr Q is a GP registrar who received a tirade of abuse from a patient, related to many longstanding issues with the practice. At the end of this phone call, Dr Q was understandably shocked and upset, and realised she was in no state to carry on with her day's work. She sought out an experienced partner in the practice, first by looking around then by knocking on doors, to request a debrief. Although there were no simple answers, this left her rejuvenated, without guilt, and enthused to try to help her next patient.

This example, while simple, could have been so different. It is only too easy to feel pressured by the list of tasks to do or patients to see. The fear of interrupting senior colleagues or of appearing weak can also be a major inhibitor. Dr Q showed considerable maturity and confidence in requesting help.

 ### *Exercise 9.1*   **Scenario**

J is an occupational therapist who has just met with a key manager, C, from the local GP commissioning consortium to discuss potential changes to the system of occupational therapy home visits locally. During the meeting, for no apparent reason, C became angry then aggressive. J was actually frightened for a short while, and although she managed to calm him down and made a swift exit, she was very shaken, particularly as she did not see it coming. Her next appointment is a visit to her team where she is expected to feedback from the previous meeting. She fears that this will be an uncomfortable meeting as her colleagues have recently been expressing strong feelings on the issue.

Exercise 9.1 (Continued)   Scenario

- What cues prior to the meeting might there have been to suggest that C may become aggressive?
- What cues during the meeting might there have been to suggest that C might become aggressive?
- What techniques might J have used to defuse the situation?
- What are the implications for the next appointment on J's schedule?
- What else might J consider to resolve the situation?
- How can she avoid this situation becoming 'entrenched'?
- Consider especially what might be driving C's behaviour.

Summary of issues

The first question J might ask herself is 'what happened there?', as there are always reasons for strong reactions. Possibly, J's attitude (even if unintentional) may have played a part. Alternatively, it may be that C's behaviour is all driven by his own situation: work or life stressors, or simply the sort of day he is having.

Going through the questions above, you might have considered the following points:

- The topic in question might have been particularly controversial; C might have a reputation for such behaviour, or the pre-meeting contact (eg emails) may have been confrontational.
- A host of non-verbal cues might have provided an early warning of irritation, eg fidgeting (or great stillness); lack of or excessive eye contact; change in body posture; increased speed or volume of speech; relative incoherence; or a refusal to answer seemingly reasonable questions. These sorts of cues are seen in all human interaction – we can use the learning we have gained from our experiences as clinicians to spot them.
- Sometimes the best thing to do is to terminate the interaction and try again at a later time. If this is not possible it may be worth considering a frank question at the first sign of trouble: 'Is there something particularly worrying you here?' or even 'Have I said something that upset you?'

- J needs to consider whether she is in the right frame of mind to go to a potentially difficult meeting, where being stressed or upset might increase the risk of a poor outcome. If not, she needs to prepare herself eg stop for a refreshment; go for a brisk walk; phone a colleague for a debrief; or find someone to talk it over with in person. If she is not prepared for the next meeting she should postpone it or try to find someone to cover her. The most professional approach may be to postpone the meeting, even if this does not sit well with her work ethic.
- One key question is whether to deal with things straight away or to 'let the dust settle' first. Remember that, however upset or angry J may feel at C's behaviour, the key is to find a solution so that her team's needs are not neglected. One of many sources of examples and advice about this question is the very readable *Fierce Conversations* (Scott, 2004).

Among the many things J might consider is the overall goal that they both share (usually better services and outcomes for patients) and how this translates into personal goals. This should enable J to connect with C and find the 'currency' he will best respond to. For example, if C is personally ambitious he may see the benefit of a project's high profile outputs, whereas if he is overwhelmed by pressures of work he may respond better to projects that will be self-running. For more detail on exchange strategies (trading what you have with what the other person desires, in exchange for what you need to accomplish your goals), it is worth looking at *Influence Without Authority* (Cohen & Bradford, 2004).

Managing yourself

Managing yourself is key to successfully managing others. Our interactions are massively affected by our state of mind and our personal feelings. There will always be difficult times in your career and how you react to these, and prevent them from affecting decisions and relationships is a key part of leadership. It is easy to underestimate that, leaders or not, clinicians are significant role models within their organisations. Their actions and attitudes are constantly looked to by colleagues. Calm, professional, respectful and supportive behaviour should be the norm, whatever the external stresses and strains.

Working with Others in primary care

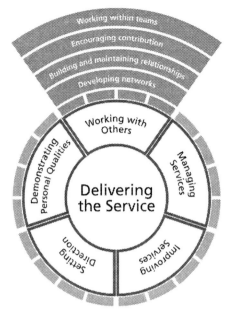

Working with others is key to clinical practice, especially in primary care. Patients in the community have a wide range of health needs that can only be met by a mixed group of professionals. Consequently both clinical practice and clinical leadership are highly dependent on these competencies.

Developing networks

One of the four elements within the *Working with Others* domain of the MLCF concerns developing networks. It is worth reflecting for a moment on the definition of a network. There are several definitions relating to computing and organisational structures, but for our purposes a network can be defined as '*an association of individuals with a common interest, formed to provide mutual support, helpful information, or the like*'. It is also interesting to remember that 'network' can be a verb: '*to cultivate people who may assist one professionally, especially in finding employment or moving to a higher position*'.

It is true that a problem shared is a problem halved. In primary care, problems come thick and fast and finding the help you need to solve them can be problematic because many clinicians work largely in isolation. Likewise, it is easy for leaders at the top of a hierarchy to become removed from their support structures or to not get advice from someone with an external perspective. Developing a functioning network is vital for survival, and while many people do it instinctively, there is always gain from some thought and self-reflection around the issue.

Consider the network of a GP working in a standard general practice. It is not completely straightforward to define this but, for argument's sake, this may include:

- Other local and national GPs
- Local GPs with special interests
- Specialist nurses
- Consultants
- Private consultants
- The community mental health team
- Pharmacist(s)
- Health visitors
- District nurses
- Macmillan nurses
- Social services
- Rapid response team
- Phlebotomists
- Key individuals from the regional health structures (eg PCT and/or SHA)
- Other practice managers
- Local Medical Committee (LMC) representatives
- BMA representatives
- Opticians

This is not an exhaustive list. However, a crucial point to note is that the GP will have formed relationships not only with the professions listed but also with these people *as individuals*. It is these relationships, and the trust that has developed, that makes this a network rather than just a long list of professionals. For example a GP may have certain district nurses who they prefer to turn to because of, for example, their above average reliability, clinical skills or availability. The nurses will probably have similar thoughts about which GPs in a practice are best to approach for specific problems.

When it comes to clinical leadership, we often think of networks as somehow different to these clinical networks, but the fundamental principle remains the same: the network you develop is based on a combination of who is available and who is likely to be helpful. Networks tend to develop opportunistically over time, dependent on day to day interactions. However, a little thought and planning can drastically improve their value. Even very senior people are susceptible to a well prepared question or compliment; these openings can then lead on to a meaningful professional relationship.

Networking

There are entire books on the art of networking, but in this section a few simple ideas are presented which can help you increase the scope and utility of your networks.

First, a problem junior clinicians often have with the concept of 'networking' is accepting the idea that they have anything to offer those senior to them. The answer to this dilemma is to consider what junior members of an organisation have that senior managers and executives may not. They might have: the time to run projects, connections to frontline staff, more recent experience in other organisations or a different awareness of patients' concerns. Second, it is worth considering who you ideally want in your network – which individuals can help you achieve your short, medium and long-term career aims?

? | ***Exercise 9.2*** | **Scenario**

P is a junior physiotherapist working in a community physiotherapy department. She would like to look at initiating innovative ways of working in the local area, and her starting point is thinking about all the different people she might want to involve. She realises the different people will have variable levels of time and energy to contribute, and have different levels of influence.

- Write a list of all the different individuals and groups that P might want to connect with.
- Are there techniques you could use to help explore the full breadth of who might want to get involved?
- How might you assess these people in terms of their levels of interest and influence?

Summary of issues

One approach to this exercise is through drawing a mindmap. There are many different web-based products that can help you

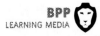

construct mindmaps of varying complexity. A very basic example of a mindmap is given in Figure 9.1.

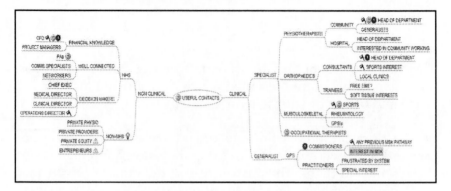

Figure 9.1 A mindmap of potential stakeholders for P the physiotherapist

Stakeholder mapping

The next step is to decide who from your longlist to target. One possible method is to rank individuals for *influence* (what they can bring to your project/career) and *interest* (how much time do they have, are they a facilitative individual etc). This can then be plotted in a 2×2 or 4×4 matrix. This is a method called stakeholder mapping which is usually applied to engagement planning, but it can also be useful in this context. More information is freely available on the internet but remember not to be too slavish in response to your rankings. In the following example, the chief executive's PA has no interest in the proposed changes, but may have a strong interest in something else you can propose. The PA's high level of *influence* (access to the chief executive's diary, for instance) may mean it is still worth investing time in the relationship. Finally, it is important to remember that a stakeholder mapping matrix is only ever a guide, and it is quite possible to alter levels of interest in colleagues through good people management and information sharing.

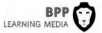

	No influence	Low influence	Moderate influence	High influence
High interest	• Entrepeneurs • Private physiotherapist			• Head of Orthopaedics • GP commissioner with interest • Responsible finance officer
Moderate interest	• Private providers	• Community physiotherapists • Occupational therapists	• GPSI • Consultants	• Clinical director
Low interest	• Private equity	• GP	• Chief Hospital physiotherapist	• CEO
No interest				• PA to CEO

Figure 9.2 Stakeholder mapping of potential stakeholders for P the physiotherapist

Building and managing relationships

Once you have established relationships with a variety of people (ie formed a network), you need to consider how to continue maintaining and using your contact list. Clearly, contacts can only be useful if you can remember who to contact and when (ie who has mutual interest in a given problem). There are several options including the old-fashioned Rolodex™ method, address book groups or a spreadsheet. A very basic example of this is included below; obviously this can be as complex and multifaceted as you like, and specialist software to constrict this is widely available.

Name	Title	Contacts	Interest	Interest
Louis Entwistle	GP local practice	Phone...	MSK medicine	Commissioning
Anna Denton	CEO, local hospital	...or email...	Integrated care	Urgent care
Emily Richardson	Management consultant	...or Skype etc.	Telehealth	Networking

Figure 9.3 A simple contact list

Another extremely popular method is through the use of a networking website. The most common one in use in the UK is LinkedIn (http://uk.linkedin.com), which gives you an easy way of establishing contact and collating details.

One final point is that maintaining a network of contacts is easier if people realise they are genuinely valued. Use of 'thank you' letters or cards, or even just an email, text or phone call to let colleagues know that you do not take their help for granted can make a huge difference. Even when you are not necessarily convinced about the value of their input it is worth appreciating the effort – you never know when you will need their help again.

Managing Services in Primary Care

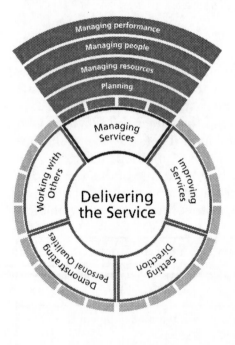

In the *Managing Services* domain of the MLCF an important element is that of 'planning'. This means actively contributing to plans to achieve service goals. At first glance this area does not necessarily correlate well with the 'day job'. By definition, general practice and most other areas of clinical practice in primary care exist as solution shops: the patient brings a problem and the doctor tries to solve it. Any planning in this process will most likely be over a short period of time during the diagnosis/early treatment phase.

Developing planning skills

There is also a chronic disease management element to primary care and this requires planning, partly for individual patients but more importantly for specific disease groups. The average GP may

Image © 2010 NHS Institute and AoMRC

only be loosely involved in the disease group management as it is often led by nursing and administrative staff. Over the next few years we are likely to see much more case management in primary care, which will require the development of new skills for many doctors.

Planning skills, useful clinically and at a practice level, will be even more important for those who get involved in commissioning. GPs and other clinicians will have a lot more influence on the strategies employed to deliver results and there will be tremendous opportunities for enthusiastic individuals to influence strategy and learn new skills.

 Exercise 9.3   **Scenario**

Dr D is a GP and a member of a new commissioning consortium. He is tasked with leading the local programme on medicines management. This year's target is to improve medicines reconciliation (the accuracy of prescriptions for patients being discharged from hospital or transferred between services). This is a huge patient safety area and it is well recognised that performance is often poor with lots of errors: one Canadian study showed discrepancies between intended and actual discharge medication lists for 41% of patients (Wong *et al.*, 2008). Dr D's consortium has found, from a small audit, that only 36% of patients are on the medications prescribed by the hospital one month after discharge.

- How should D approach this problem?
- What strategies and tools might he consider using to improve the current situation?

Summary of issues

It is beyond the scope of this chapter to give you a complete plan for tackling this longstanding problem, which encompasses complex systems and a wide range of stakeholders. Instead, the list below is a brief synopsis of potential methods you can use to make improvements, which are followed by a more detailed review of process mapping.

Improvement methodologies

More improvement methodologies are described in other chapters, and all are widely available from online sources such as the NHS Institute of Innovation and Improvement website (www.institute. nhs.uk).

- **Data:** one of the key issues facing the NHS is data availability and quality; how do you know what the problem is and how will you know if you are improving it? This is not necessarily captured in standard clinical systems and may need a new approach. Use your networks to find people who can help you understand the problem and find a solution.

- **Process mapping:** if you want to change the system you need to know what the current processes are before you can suggest improvements. Process mapping basically means 'walking through' all the current steps, ideally by actually going to where they happen. In Exercise 9.3 Dr D might visit the hospital pharmacy, the ward, the patient's home, their local pharmacy and the GP surgery. A process such as medicines reconciliation is likely to be managed in different ways by different practices and pharmacies, so standardisation has significant potential benefits in terms of safety and efficiency.

- **Root cause analysis:** this methodology is focused on attempting to understand where errors come from, and subsequently identifying and prioritising areas where improvements could be made.

- **Feedback:** the most valuable resource at your disposal is the users of the current system, ie patients (the 'end-users'), commissioners (the people who 'buy' services) and staff. This resource is often neglected when planning new services; a few simple questions could probably identify areas of improvement. One method of obtaining this, covered in other chapters in this book, is multi-source feedback.

- **Driver diagrams:** a way of generating change hypotheses. This is a form of brainstorming which produces multiple hypotheses that can then be tested. Clinical leaders (as well as service users) with their front-line experience have a critical role in explaining what will work, and what will not, when it comes to implementing ideas.

- **PDSA cycles:** perhaps the best way to make and test changes, the PDSA (Plan-Do-Study-Act) cycle is a simple model which allows busy people with multiple commitments to make incremental improvements to a service. Unlike audit, PDSAs may be run very frequently eg daily or weekly with small changes each time (NHS Institute of Innovation and Improvement, 2011).

Process mapping

As mentioned above, process mapping is a method for understanding the steps involved in a process so that it might be improved. Maps range from the simple to the highly complex. The overall goal is to simplify the process as much as possible into lots of single steps, to reduce variation and maximise efficiency. There are also situations where it may be advantageous to break the map down into subsections – this is called block process mapping. Examples of process mapping might include reorganising supplies to make everything available reliably at the place they will be needed, or agreeing a series of steps that will constitute local policy.

Value stream mapping

Another way of approaching the same problem is value stream mapping, which was developed by the Toyota car company. This is essentially the same as process mapping but separates out key parts of the process – the 'value adding' steps – from those more to do with 'preparing for' or 'cleaning up after' those steps. One other slight difference is an emphasis on the flow of materials during any pathway, which led to the idea of 'just-in-time' material provision (ordering small, exact quantities of stock, rather than keeping huge supplies and bulk-buying).

The classic process map used for illustration is how to make a cup of tea (an important *housekeeping* skill!). Try this for yourself, then apply the same approach to Dr D's medicines reconciliation problem mentioned above or a current service issue within your department. To keep it simple, try to think in terms of only two different types of step and keep the map on one page:

- Process – a step or activity
- Decision – usually a yes/no option with appropriate branches

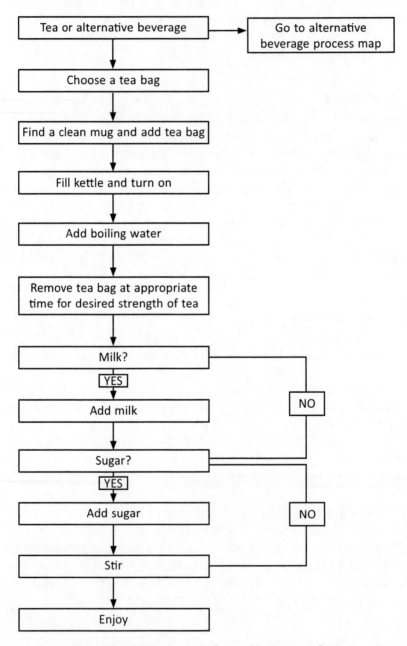

Figure 9.4 A process map for making a cup of tea

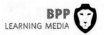

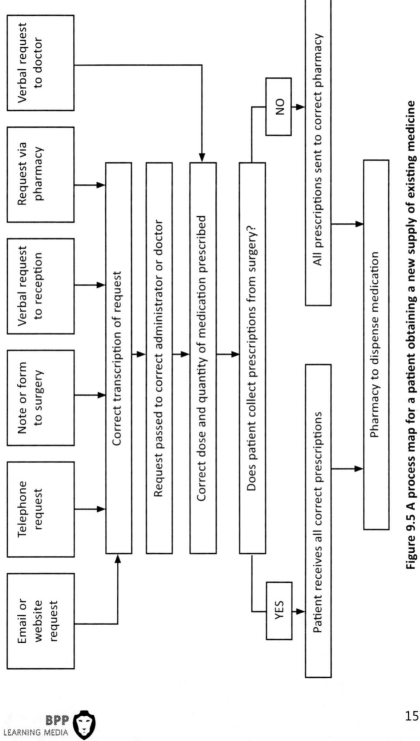

Figure 9.5 A process map for a patient obtaining a new supply of existing medicine

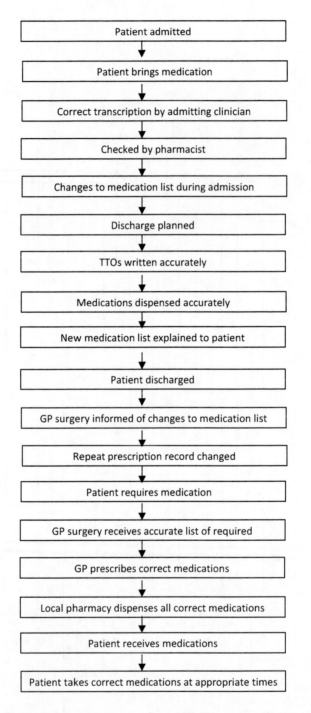

Figure 9.6 A process map for medicines reconciliation

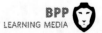

Improving Services in Primary Care

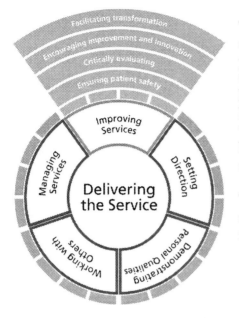

This section relates to a key art of management: motivating your workforce to work towards a joint vision. In UK healthcare, despite the NHS being one of the strongest 'brands' in the world, this has been surprisingly difficult to achieve across the board.

The MLCF refers to four key components that together facilitate transformation:

- Model the change expected
- Articulate the need for change and its impact on people and services
- Promote changes leading to systems redesign
- Motivate and focus a group to accomplish change

Involving colleagues to accomplish change

Successful transformation requires a degree of all of these components, and without doubt motivation and focus are vital qualities for any group embarking on change. This process of engagement can be described in five key stages (NHS London, 2010):

1. **Status:** what is the current state of engagement?
2. **Plan:** how will people react to change and how can you deal with their reactions?
3. **Target:** which groups do you need to prioritise for engagement?
4. **Involve:** draw people into the change process so that they feel part of it

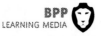

5.   **Act:** get the change started and ensure it runs as smoothly as possible

Although each stage is important, this chapter has particular focus on the *involve* stage. There is strong evidence that *involved* staff and patients – which can be measured quantitatively using the Medical Engagement Scale developed by Peter Spurgeon and colleagues (Spurgeon, Barwell and Mazelan, 2011) – will *engage* with the process of care, and help deliver far superior outcomes. This is true for day-to-day-work (for a succinct explanation of this as an argument see *The Meaning of Careful* [Brown, 2009]), but it is particularly important for change. If engagement is neglected the best laid plans can come to nothing.

Clinical engagement

The principle of *clinical engagement* is often referred to in healthcare management, yet experience tells us that it is much neglected both in primary and secondary care. The NHS has huge untapped potential in its workforce; unleashing this depends upon concentrating on what makes people tick. The reason that *clinical* engagement is given a higher profile than *staff* engagement is probably to do with the unique perspective of frontline clinicians, their regular contact with patients, and the insights they bring to strategic change. However, the principles can and should be applied across the healthcare workforce.

The clinical engagement ladder

This clinical engagement ladder is adapted from Arnstein's *Ladder of Citizen Engagement* (Arnstein, 1969). It is intended as an aid to help consider why people behave in the ways they do and which groups need the most input, and when. The ladder reflects how engagement levels vary between individuals over time. Clearly the divisions between sections are arbitrary; in reality this is a continuum with multiple shades of grey rather than a binary of black and white.

Status	Engagement level	Tactics
Actively engaged	Leading Involved	• Support leadership development • Sufficient status • Maintain strong support • Remuneration
Passively engaged	Influential Aligned	• Seek to involve • Target key individuals to become champions
Danger point	Activated (Positive or negative)	• Focused communications • Face to face time • Active listening
Disengaged	Informed Unaware	• Generalised communications • Work with the press • Get to know

Figure 9.7 The clinical engagement ladder

It is hard to argue against helping people climb the ladder as a positive thing – the more informed and interested our clinical workforce is, the easier it is to improve quality. There is debate over whether to aim to develop everyone or just a specific cadre to the 'actively engaged' stage, but in most cases this is usually likely to be a self-selecting group.

The danger of disengagement

A potential danger point is 'activation', where people receive more and more information and form opinions about it. Given that change often excites strong reactions and can be controversial, there is a danger of ending up with misalignment, which can lead to individuals who are actively *disengaged*. This can be quite a comfortable position for many clinicians with respect to change programmes (eg the BMA response to the 2010 Health White Paper), as it protects the status quo and often plays well with the profession and the public. It is possible to think of this as a parallel ladder of clinical *disengagement*.

This group, in the 'activated' section of the ladder, therefore requires special thought and effort. In particular, it is important not to ignore their concerns. The focus should instead be on trying to provide answers one by one and sticking to the principles of the project, even if the debate becomes heated or messy.

Core messages

There are many other topics relevant to clinical engagement, but for reasons of space, we will look at just one more: the generation of core messages.

 Exercise 9.4   **Scenario**

Dr W is an inner city GP. Her finance director (FD) has approached her to ask for help in engaging the local GPs and district nurses. There is a plan to move them all into a new Private Finance Initiative (PFI) building to save a million pounds a year in overheads and maintenance costs. The FD has been stung by the negative reaction he has had from a few GPs so far.

- What messages can you think of that would play well to this audience?
- What methods could W use to get this message across?

Summary of issues

It may be a mistake for Dr W to assume a financial argument will not be challenged. This neglects a host of other factors. In this example, the GPs and district nurses are likely to have sentimental attachments to their current sites; concerns about the inconvenience of moving; potential personality clashes with colleagues from different teams; anxiety about their current premises (which the GPs may own and earn income from) or parking arrangements... the list goes on. Some of these concerns may be universal, others may be specific to local circumstance.

Leaders need to try to pre-empt these understandable human feelings and to tailor their messages appropriately. The following points may help:

- Clinicians usually respond best to arguments about clinical quality or patient experience.
    - Use evidence where possible to make the case for change.
    Is there any negative patient feedback about current buildings? Have there been any safety issues?
    - Focus on the patient and the benefits of a new, healthcare-specific building, which may be in terms of service quality or patient experience.
    Is there any evidence from any similar projects elsewhere?
- Financial imperatives may be best left tacit as they become mixed up with individual concerns about income, job security etc.
    - If talking about money, emphasise the benefits to patients and clinicians of freeing up resources for new or improved services.
    If possible give examples, with modelling of the projected benefits. There may also be, for example, an environmental argument such as the new building being carbon-neutral. Again use data where possible: try to show the waste in the current system.
- Try to find positives to 'sell' the idea.
    - Do not try for too many and make sure you can back them up.
    The parking may actually be better in the new site; communication between teams may be facilitated; there may be better relaxation facilities for staff; the site may be more convenient for travel etc.

A discussion of the best methods for getting these messages out could fill a whole book. However, to summarise, the absolute key is to 'front-up'. Even if the audience is going to be difficult, it is crucial to apply active listening whilst also sticking clearly to your core messages. People's minds will only be put at rest if you actually address their concerns or help them believe that the alternatives are better. This is about integrity. *This is leadership*!

Setting Direction in primary care

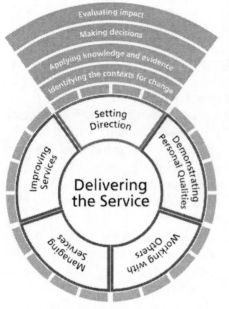

As detailed in other chapters a key element of the MLCF *Setting Direction* domain involves applying knowledge and evidence. This entails:

- Using appropriate methods to gather data and information
- Undertaking analysis against an evidence-based criteria set
- Using information to challenge existing practices and processes
- Influencing others to use knowledge and evidence to achieve best practice

Evidence-based service improvement

Evidence-based medicine (EBM) is now an accepted part of clinical practice: EBM skills are widely taught; national and local guidelines exist for most clinical conditions; and clinicians regularly question the evidence base for proposed changes (see Chapter 7 and the use of BestBETS in the Emergency Department). It is, however, easy to confuse two issues here. Most people would accept the premise that clinical decision-making should be, where possible, based on evidence. However, it is much harder to base service improvement on an evidence base. This is because there is generally less evidence available (there may be evidence for the clinical steps in a pathway but not for the organisational structures) Additionally, health systems are inherently complex, so assumptions must be made about whether changes made in one area can be extrapolated to another.

 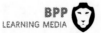

Exercise 9.5 (part a)   Scenario

Dr R is a recently qualified salaried GP in a large practice, where the current system of diabetes management is achieving poor results, poor patient and staff satisfaction and relatively long waiting times. The partners in the practice ask Dr R to look at how to improve the service. She knows they are concerned about the financial implications of the current poor service both for themselves and the local health economy and she hopes to impress them with her strategic and managerial skills. Dr R also knows that NICE recently updated its diabetes guidance and she wants to implement this.

- What possible approaches can you think of that Dr R can use for developing her strategy to implement NICE guidance?
- Do not worry about what the strategy will be, just try to think of as many options as possible for formulating it.

Summary of issues

Formulating a well-planned strategy for improving the diabetic service through the implementation of the NICE guidance, could take a number of different approaches, including:

- Interpret the NICE guidance and draw up changes
- Ask GP colleagues for their opinions
- Ask the practice nurses and receptionists how the system could be improved
- Ask the local diabetologists for their opinions
- Ask another local practice how they manage diabetes
- Look nationally for exemplars eg through Map of Medicine, your Strategic Health Authority, the Department of Health, the press, health charities etc
- Look internationally for impressive service models
- Group up with your local consortium to design a service across all the local practices

When planning services, pragmatic decisions may need to be made. It may not be possible to ensure the evidence for a particular proposal is directly relevant to the local circumstances and patient population, and in this situation the decision may have to be a 'best guess'.

 Exercise 9.5 (part b)   **Scenario**

Dr R is then asked to develop the new diabetes service model for the local commissioning consortium, and decides to base it on the care planning approach developed by Diabetes UK. This will require considerable changes in working methods for some local practices and she anticipates some dissent.

- How might Dr R present the ideas to colleagues in local practices?
- Think specifically about how she could use the evidence base to make her case.

Summary of issues

There are a number of strategies that may help Dr R to build a case for change, and encourage her colleagues to support her proposals. These approaches might include:

- Exploring whether or not there is a problem with existing practice.
    - Utilise the Quality and Outcomes Framework and any other data she might have available (eg Secondary Uses Service data from the local hospital) to shine a light on current performance.
    - Show the practices (privately) how they compare to their peers on markers of good practice.
    - If no local practices perform well, find 'beacon' data from a similar area elsewhere in the country to show what is possible.
    - Look for evidence of patient safety episodes around diabetes and discuss these.
- Involve clinical champions.
    - Get as many local and national clinicians behind her model as possible and try to use their support and influence at meetings. If the project was being led by a manager, it would be particularly helpful to use clinical champions to deliver key messages at meetings.

  – Specify the desired (evidence-based) *outcomes* and let the 'locals', which ideally would include clinicians, managers and patients, design the *process* which will deliver them.

To summarise, there is no doubt that change should be evidence-based wherever possible. However, it may be that the evidence extends only to the best surrogate outcomes (eg the target HbA1c or blood pressure in diabetics) or to certain steps in the process (eg patient education). Strong leadership is essential in order to design an efficient system that does not alienate the key participants.

Summary

Leadership in general practice is needed more than ever, both at micro (the practice) and macro (commissioning consortium, LMC, RCGP, commissioning board etc) levels. Just as importantly, knowing when to demonstrate *followership* is a key part of leadership; even the most senior leaders recognise when to put their weight behind someone else's project or campaign.

The examples presented in this chapter give a sense – the tip of the iceberg – of the immense number of exciting leadership challenges and development opportunities available for junior clinicians in general practice. If you feel these are hidden to you, seek one out, because there is often a snowball effect where a small project can soon develop into more offers of work than you can reasonably manage (which is when you will need to develop the crucial skill of saying 'no' to things). If you are struggling with this, use your networking skills to find a senior clinician or manager who can mentor you and help you identify opportunities.

Finally, this chapter and, indeed, this book give you a framework for thinking about how to develop your skills and career. This is a great thing. However, there are two key caveats. First, do not neglect the wider leadership literature as many leadership skills are generic and, second, do not be afraid to try out things even if they don't completely fit your career plan. Career development is like surfing. If you see a wave (an opportunity) you think might be fun, or interesting or useful, then ride it for a bit.

If it doesn't work out look for the next wave – there will be another one along any minute.

Three things to try

1. Find a problem area within your practice – perhaps a prescribing or QoF target that you are not meeting, or something a patient may have mentioned to you. Try drawing a process map to show you what happens under the current system and highlight the problem areas. What would a better process map look like?
2. Map out your personal network. Think about which people you would approach with different kinds of problems. Next time you are planning a change – perhaps in response to your process map – think hard about who can help you implement it and what 'currency' (how you should present the information and what you can offer them) you need to use to encourage them to help you.
3. Consider how you might engage the staff within your organisation with either their day-to-day work or a change programme you are instigating. Where do they sit on the engagement ladder? How can you avoid them becoming actively disengaged? What key messages do you need to get across to different groups and how will you go about doing this? How will you know if you are succeeding?

References

Arnstein, Sherry R. A Ladder of Citizen Participation. *JAIP* 1969; Vol. 35, No. 4, July: 216–224.

British Medical Association. *Resources for Doctors in Difficulty* (June 2011) [Online] Available at www.bma.org.uk/doctors_health/d4dresourcesfordoctorsindifficulty.jsp [Accessed 17/10/11].

British Medical Association. *Doctors Health Matters: A report by the Health Policy & Economic Research Unit, 2007* [Online] Available at www.bma.org.uk/doctors_health/doctorshealth.jsp [Accessed 17/10/11].

Brown DJ (2009) *The Meaning of Careful: How Putting People Before Process Will Deliver Outstanding Results and Transform Our Healthcare.* London: HCV Publishing.

Cohen AR and Bradford DL (2005) *Influence Without Authority.* US: Wiley.

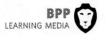

Neighbour R (2005) *The Inner Consultation: How to Develop an Effective and Intuitive Consulting Style*. Oxford: Radcliffe Publishing.

NHS Institute of Innovation and Improvement. *Plan Do Study Act toolkit* [Online] Available at www.institute.nhs.uk/quality_and_service_improvement_tools/quality_and_service_improvement_tools/plan_do_study_act.html [Accessed 17/10/11].

NHS Institute of Innovation and Improvement. *Process mapping – an overview* [Online] Available at www.institute.nhs.uk/quality_and_service_improvement_tools/quality_and_service_improvement_tools/process_mapping_-_an_overview.html [Accessed 17/10/11].

NHS London. *Engagement Handbook* [Online] Available at www.london.nhs.uk/webfiles/Communications/Strategic%20Plans%20MP/HANDBOOK%20all%20sections%20FINAL%20eVERSION%20August%202010.pdf [Accessed 17/10/11].

Scott S (2004) *Fierce Conversations Achieving Success in Work and in Life, One Conversation at a Time.* New York, US: Berkley Publishing Group.

Spurgeon P, Barwell F and Mazelan P. Medical Engagement: A crucial underpinning to organizational performance. *Health Serv Manager Res* 2011; 24(3): 114–120.

Wong JD *et al*. Medication Reconciliation at Hospital Discharge: Evaluating Discrepancies. *The Annals of Pharmacotherapy* 2008; 42(10): 1373–1379.

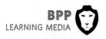

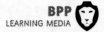

Chapter 10

Leadership Learning as an Undergraduate

Katie de Wit &
Bob Klaber

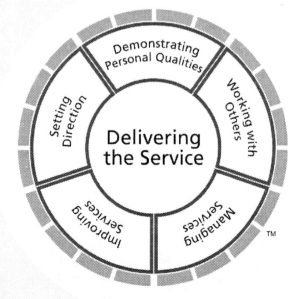

Leadership Learning as an Undergraduate

 ### *Chapter overview*

This chapter examines the opportunities for leadership learning as an undergraduate, and explores a number of key concepts including:

- Taking on a role as a patient 'advocate'
- Role-modelling
- Groupthink
- Learning about financial flows within the health service
- Moving beyond audit to improve care
- Measuring quality through patient experience measures
- The role of students and doctors in promoting sustainable healthcare

 This chapter also looks at practical tools and techniques which can be used to support learning. These include:

- SBAR to aid communication
- The WHO surgical checklist
- Work shadowing
- Audit cycles and PDSA cycles
- PROMs (Patient-Reported Outcome Measures) as a marker of patient experience

---

Introduction

What it means to be a doctor is changing, with more than just clinical excellence needed to provide high quality care to patients. As medical school is where we learn the foundations of how to be a good doctor, it is important that learning focuses on *all* the attributes of being a good doctor. This includes learning to be a competent leader in the NHS. The GMC guidance in *Tomorrow's Doctors* is beginning to reflect this reality and the MLCF Undergraduate Guidance sets out the knowledge, behaviours, skills and attitudes that are appropriate and achievable at undergraduate level.

Initially it may be difficult to see the opportunities for medical students to develop their leadership and management skills. Suggestions have traditionally been met with a cry of 'but I'm just a medical student, what can I do?' In reality, however, there are many opportunities to gain this experience. Some are easy to find, others require more proactive behaviours during the clinical years of undergraduate training. Medical students have specific attributes and hold a unique position in the eyes of the patient, which means they are well placed to play an (often under-used) important role in hospitals and GP surgeries. Taking this role on not only helps improve care for the patient but also helps develop their own leadership and management skills. Becoming more involved can also transform medical students' experiences of placements, moving them from the perception of being a spare part, always in the way and not being particularly useful, to feeling like a valued member of the team.

First, medical students often have an abundance of time, and in particular, time with patients to explore their ideas, concerns and expectations. There are often circumstances where doctors do not have the time to do this, which can be a missed opportunity; exploring these areas can have a major influence on a patient's care. Students can also help patients prepare for ward rounds or consultations with their GP so that they can make the most out of their time with the consultant / registrar / GP. Although often an understandable frustration for medical students, not being seen as a 'proper' member of the medical team has its advantages for patients, who can see the medical student as a different sort of advocate in their care. For example, medical students can help guide patients on their journey through hospital, which can be a confusing and frightening experience. What is more, medical students can act as 'fresh eyes' on practice. Are things done differently / better / more efficiently in other GP practices or wards or hospitals? Medical students, who move around every few weeks and are not yet indoctrinated into a fixed way of doing things, may bring innovative ideas or a new perspective on an old problem.

Making the most of the years in medical school requires three things: an appreciation of the importance and relevance of these skills to being a doctor; an awareness of the opportunities available; and an enthusiastic, proactive nature and willingness to take advantage of them. The first requirement is dealt with throughout this book and the last is down to the individual medical student. This chapter uses the domains of the MLCF to illustrate the second: a wide, but by no means exhaustive, range of opportunities that are available to students.

Demonstrating Personal Qualities as an undergraduate

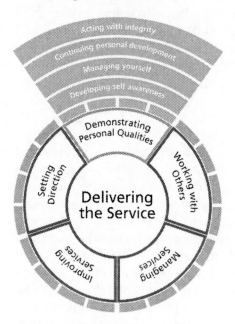

Demonstrating Personal Qualities is an obvious starting point for medical students to explore ideas around self-awareness and their approach to learning and development. An example of this is through adopting role models.

Role-modelling

Role-modelling has traditionally been an informal way to instil the professional values of medicine in medical students as they progress through the medical hierarchy. Studies have shown that medical students look for enthusiasm, compassion, openness, integrity, and good relationships with patients in their role models (Paice *et al.*, 2002). Interestingly, the same studies show that students are not yet choosing to model themselves on those in senior management roles, service development and professional leadership positions. This perhaps reflects both the historical lack of emphasis on these attributes within medicine as a profession, and the lack of exposure to those who are involved in these activities.

Although it is impossible for students to choose who to surround themselves with on placements, all experiences of senior colleagues,

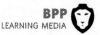

whether positive or negative, can provide useful learning. While there are certainly common attributes to most good leaders, there is not one model of leadership that suits every personality type or situation (Patel *et al.*, 2010). Effective leaders can adapt their leadership style to the person or people being influenced, as well as the task or goal at hand. One of the bonuses of medical school is the sheer volume of clinicians and other healthcare workers students encounter throughout their studies. When on placements, it is worth watching, and thinking about, how different doctors react in different scenarios:

- How do they deal with stressful situations?
- How do they chair multidisciplinary team (MDT) meetings or break bad news?
- What supportive or difficult behaviours do they exhibit?

The influence of role models, whether positive or negative, on how medical students and junior doctors develop cannot be underestimated. Role-modelling can mean that professional values and attitudes are difficult to change from generation to generation. Some have suggested a divergence in the qualities that medical students say they admire and those that they actually emulate in practice. There is a danger of 'personal ideals waning' as they become immersed further into the profession, and then go on to subconsciously adopt the behaviours of those around them. Studies have shown students who had witnessed unethical behaviour in their consultants were also more likely to report doing something unethical themselves (Paice *et al.*, 2002).

Therefore, it is important that role-modelling is an active, reflective process rather than a passive, absorptive one. A simple exercise to demonstrate this process and identify areas for development is explained in Figure 10.1.

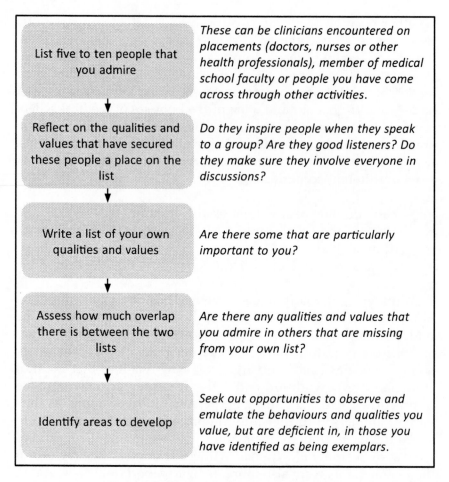

Figure 10.1 Reflecting on your role models

Becoming more aware of role modelling, including on how people may look at you, and actively reflecting on the attitudes and behaviours of those around you is a good way to develop yourself. Developing informal or formal mentoring relationships with role models can also be a very successful and fulfilling method of personal and professional development. A successful mentoring relationship will also bring benefits to the mentor (Warren and Carnall, 2010).

Working with Others as an undergraduate

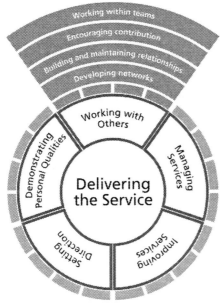

This section builds on the discussions around self development and role-modelling to explore how individual attitudes and behaviours impact on teamworking.

Understanding teamworking

As healthcare becomes ever more complex in the way it is organised and delivered, high quality care and patient safety relies on team members continually gathering and sharing knowledge. A poorly organised or dysfunctional team can have dire consequences for patients. As a medical student, it is worth taking some time to think about what makes a good team opposed to a poor one, and exploring what roles one can play in them. This is illustrated in the exercise below.

 ### *Exercise 10.1*   Scenario

Having started on her care of the elderly ward, Susie, a fourth year medical student, was surprised at how many different types of clinicians and other care professions were involved in the care of each patient. It felt very different from other placements that she had been on where she felt the doctors seemed to be more 'in charge'. Susie mentioned this to her consultant, who encouraged her to explore how the team worked together over the course of the placement, and to give her reflections on this during her end of placement assessment.

- How might Susie explore the roles of different specialties and professions?
- How might she evaluate the quality of the teamwork?

Summary of issues

There are different ways in which she could achieve this. For example, Susie might also like to evaluate information flows between members, to see whether communication is timely with adequate information handed over. There are various frameworks to guide patient-related communication between healthcare workers, such as Situation-Background-Assessment-Recommendation (SBAR), which was discussed in detail in Chapter 6. This allows each member to focus their information, and facilitates shared expectations on what should be communicated and how it should be done. It might also be interesting for Susie to explore how the team interact with their patients. Do their patients understand the roles of each person looking after them? How effectively does each member of the team communicate with them? Is there unnecessary duplication of tasks?

Susie could spend time with each member of the MDT prior to a weekly MDT meeting. She could then see what information each member gathers and inputs into the meeting. She could also evaluate how the meeting is run. Does everybody have a chance to input? Is there a diversity of contributions, or does the consultant make the decision and the rest of the team agree without thought? Does this differ between consultants?

Groupthink

Susie's experience of an MDT might also have revealed the phenomenon of groupthink. Groupthink is the process of decision-making within highly cohesive groups, characterised by uncritical acceptance or conformity (Janis, 1982). Without value being placed on diversity of opinion and input, teams are at best not reaching their potential, and at worst unsafe. Medical students, in their lowly status in the medical hierarchy, and often undervalued in teams, are particularly susceptible to developing a 'groupthink' mentality. For example, in one US study, 76% of medical students said they had witnessed an error on the wards, but only half of them reported the incident. 'Complexity theory' emphasises that diversity in the way team members gather and process information is essential, so that while cohesiveness is a laudable aim of a healthcare team, an element of constructive challenge is necessary.

Encouraging, listening to and valuing dissenting opinion may be the most important characteristic of teams that act in a patient's best interest. That a team member is able to speak up so that clinical error is avoided before it has fatal consequences is vital. So is the ability to speak against a prevailing ethical view. Apparent consensus is not always the best defence against unethical decision-making.

(Snelgrove *et al.*, 2010)

Teamworking in theatres: the WHO surgical checklist

Surgical theatres are a particularly good place for medical students to observe and reflect on good and poor team dynamics. As a busy, pressured and multidisciplinary environment, the operating theatre provides the perfect environment for unclear communication, clashing motivations and ultimately errors. Surgery is also quite a hierarchical specialty, with a traditional view that still persists in certain areas of a lone surgeon relying on their courage, wits, experience and improvisation to save the patient. This can mean that there is a danger that those lower down the team hierarchy do not have a genuine voice. Indeed, in the majority of so-called 'never events' in surgery (for example, operating on the wrong limb), someone in the team knew something was wrong but felt unable to speak up, or if they were, they went unheard (Michaels *et al.*, 2007).

As described in Chapter 8, the World Health Organization (WHO) Surgical Safety Checklist, introduced in 2009, was designed specifically to create *'an atmosphere of mutual trust in which all staff members can talk freely about safety problems and how to solve them, without fear of blame or punishment'* (Institute of Healthcare Improvement, 2011). As observers in theatre, students can watch how the team (who may well have not worked together before) goes through the surgical checklist. How influential is this process? Is the checklist helping create such a culture, or is the team using it purely as an enforced tick-box exercise, with little impact on the team dynamics?

Managing Services as an Undergraduate

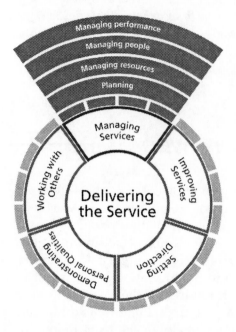

Part of effective leadership in the NHS is showing a responsibility to ensure the success of the organisation where you work. The NHS will only thrive if its resources, including the people who work within it, are deployed and managed effectively. This does not mean that every doctor should take on a formal management role, but the knowledge, skills, behaviours and attitudes involved in managing services are relevant in the day-to-day duties of all doctors.

It is only by understanding how NHS services are planned, funded and evaluated that doctors can hope to make an active contribution in the improvement of healthcare delivery. Their awareness of how the NHS is resourced, and the ability to use their influence as a doctor to ensure resources are used appropriately, will ensure that more of the needs of their patients and the wider community can be met. Traditionally, this has not been seen as priority learning and medical schools have been slow to emphasise it in their curricula. Consequently, most medical students have a poor awareness of the importance of planning and managing resources, people and performance.

Learning about financial flows in primary care

Gaining experience of managing services in the NHS as a medical student requires a proactive approach, as this aspect of healthcare has traditionally been kept separate from clinicians. GPs operate as 'small businesses' and so primary care placements are a good place to start. With many GPs taking on a lead role in clinical commissioning groups, their role in commissioning services and

Image © 2010 NHS Institute and AoMRC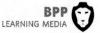

managing resources for their local population will significantly increase. Asking a GP or practice manager to talk about the impact of cost considerations, commissioning and funding streams in primary care can lead to valuable insights. Students can look at how a surgery is performing on the Quality and Outcomes Framework, through which they are partially funded (The Information Centre, 2011) and can then ask their GP about how this affects the planning and development of services. There may be opportunities to find out how the practice is staffed and how professionals are performance managed, and it may be possible to explore some of the relationships the practice has with local acute or mental health providers. How are services commissioned and paid for? What are the mechanisms for ensuring that patients are given the highest possible quality of care?

Shadowing as an undergraduate

Students on hospital placements can look out for any changes in hospital policies, such as the implementation of a new rota, or handover system. Why was the policy changed and how was this change managed? Was the change in policy piloted first? By talking to staff, students can get an idea of the impact of these policy changes. Medical students do not normally get much or any exposure to hospital management, but shadowing can be an excellent way to get a flavour of the role of hospital managers. This may be through spending time with a service manager or general manager, or equally through shadowing a senior nurse (eg one of the ward managers) or clinician (eg a clinical lead) as they fulfil some of their management duties. By having a clear idea of what one wants to get out of the shadowing (for example, an overview of daily activities, an idea of how managers and clinicians interact, or some insight into how policies are planned), the person being shadowed will be able to choose appropriate times and activities for a student to join them.

Improving Services as an undergraduate

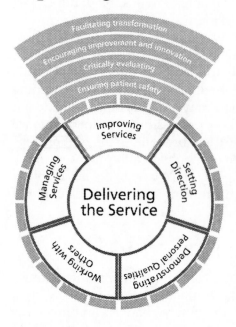

As doctors take on more responsibility for improving the quality of NHS services, and not just for the individual care they deliver, medical students should see this as an integral part of their learning during their clinical placements. This learning can come through identifying risks to patients and taking responsibility for minimising these risks. For instance, on the ward round, a student could make it their responsibility to check whether all patients have had their DVT risk assessments.

They could research common prescribing errors and drug interactions and look out for these on drug charts, or they could make sure that patients at risk of falls have everything within reach and there are no potential hazards around their beds. When writing in the notes a student could double check all patient notes have the correct basic information on every page. These are simple interventions that can have a noticeable impact on the quality of care for patients.

Moving beyond audit

Audits are always happening somewhere in a hospital, and it is relatively easy to take on a role in these. Well thought out audit projects, that have a clear question, senior supervision and approval can be a powerful way to improve patient care, as well as being a useful learning experience. However, although audit is a valuable method of ensuring that acceptable standards are being reached, they are a retrospective analysis and do not necessarily mean that the care will ultimately be improved as a result. Frustratingly, large numbers of audits do not get beyond the data collection stage and hence do not result in any change or improvement to patient care (Dharamshi, 2011).

Image © 2010 NHS Institute and AoMRC

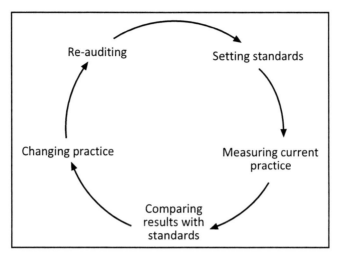

Figure 10.2 The audit cycle

Increasing numbers of medical students are developing their own quality improvement projects which they can plan and lead themselves. There are simple methodologies such as the PDSA (Plan, Do, Study, Act) cycle, described in Chapter 9, which can provide a framework for improvement.

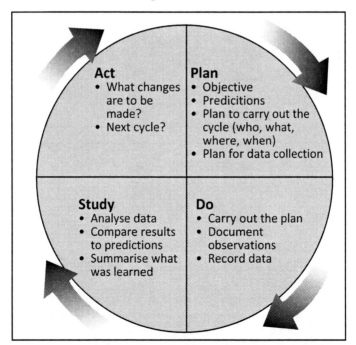

Figure 10.3 The PDSA cycle

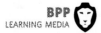

Following a PDSA cycle allows change to be planned, tested on a small scale, assessed, improved upon and trialled again before full implementation (NHS Institute for Innovation and Improvement, 2008).

Improving patient experience

'High quality care', means care that is not only effective but also safe, efficient, timely, offers value for money and is personal (Darzi, 2008). Patient experience is now becoming a key marker of quality in the NHS, with clinical outcome measures incorporating the patient to a greater degree through patient-reported outcome measures (PROMs). Furthermore, there is evidence that patient experiences directly affect outcomes (Little *et al.*, 2001). Improving services is not about simply maximising the clinical quality of care, but enhancing the experience of patients while they are interact with the healthcare system. Medical students have time to develop good rapport with patients and explore their experiences in depth. They have the freedom to be able to see and follow the whole patient journey, rather than just experience the specific intervention points (that are the only aspects of care many doctors see during their clinical work).

Exercise 10.2   **Scenario**

During a respiratory placement, Peter's consultant told him that the Trust was not scoring very highly on patient experience measures. Peter wanted to get a better appreciation of why this might be. He therefore decided to follow a patient through the system, from their acute presentation in A&E, spending time with them on the respiratory ward, right the way through to their discharge. Throughout this time, Peter focused on finding out:

- What are the factors that make a difference to patient's experience?
- How does this compare with how things are done at other hospitals?
- What can the hospital do that will improve these things?

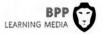

Summary of issues

The exercise of following a patient through their 'journey' in hospital is an extremely powerful way of understanding the patient perspective. As discussed in Chapter 9 there is also the opportunity to process map the different steps involved for the patient; this can lead to a greater understanding of the value (or not) of each of the steps. However, there is potential for medical students to go further than Peter does in Exercise 10.2. The divide between primary care and secondary care can often lead to disjointed care for patients. Experiencing the entire journey with a patient across these organisational boundaries has the potential to highlight the specific problems the patient experiences. Most medical schools now have community or GP placements relating to each specialty. It may be possible to follow a specific patient from their initial presentation to the GP, through their tests (in primary or secondary care), their consultation and intervention in secondary or tertiary care and their follow-up back in the community. This experience can give a student a unique 'patient-eye' view of the NHS, highlighting exactly where inefficiencies, poor handover of care and ultimately poor patient experiences occur.

Medical students can help improve services through qualitative research. This uses methodology from the social sciences to unpick trends previously highlighted by quantitative methods. Many wards have hand-held computers that collect data on whether patients have had a good or bad experience, and can track progress over time. However, these types of surveys are very restricted in their scope. Qualitative research allows patients to set the agenda and reflect on what is important to them. Although this research method requires more effort to collect and analyse data, it gives richer information than answering closed questions on aspects of care that we think are most important.

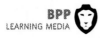

Setting Direction as an undergraduate

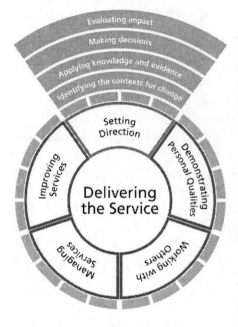

As a medical student it is easy to be sheltered from the wider context in which the NHS operates. However, political, ethical and legal factors have as much influence as purely clinical factors on how and why the NHS operates the way that it does. For example, in addition to the traditional model of a consultation (presenting complaint, history of presenting complaint, past medical history, and so on) a GP consultation is influenced by the Department of Health QoF indicators. Similarly, where people go for their minor operations (the hospital, an independent treatment centre or even their GP practice) is determined not only by clinical factors but also by government policies such as patient choice, the move towards 'care closer to home', commissioning decisions and financial considerations. It is important for medical students to understand why these decisions are made. They are not the natural evolution of healthcare, but often deliberate policies made in a particular social context.

Learning about the wider context

There are many free organisations and e-newsletters that can help medical students stay abreast of key issues and policies. The Network (www.the-network.org.uk) is a free membership organisation for medical students and junior doctors interested in leadership and management. It sends a monthly e-newsletter with a summary of interesting events, blogs and discussions. Young Civitas for Medics (www.ycfm.org.uk) hosts a series of debates in London on pertinent issues in healthcare. BMA news and the Student BMJ (www.student. bmj.com) are also good sources of up-to-date information, as are many of the Medical Royal College websites. The King's Fund

Image © 2010 NHS Institute and AoMRC

and the Nuffield Trust are two independent bodies that publish extensively on contemporary health policy issues; each have a number of well written resources available on their websites.

Sustainable healthcare

Gaining experience of setting direction in the NHS can be difficult for medical students. With a bit of imagination, it is possible to identify areas where medical students can contribute to the formulation of strategy. One example might be a hospital's undergraduate teaching programme. Another good example is in the area of 'sustainable healthcare'. The Climate Change Act 2008 legally obliges NHS organisations to take action to reduce carbon dioxide equivalent emissions by 80% by 2050, with an interim target of a 10% reduction by 2015 (NHS Sustainable Development Unit, 2010). However, this concept has not yet become mainstream in the consciousness of most NHS staff, and therefore provides an arena for the younger generation of healthcare professionals to drive forward an awareness of the environmental and social impacts of the NHS. This in turn provides an excellent opportunity for medical students to get involved in helping decide strategies, as shown in Exercise 10.3.

Exercise 10.3   Scenario

Melanie is a medical student on a general placement at a GP surgery. She is given the impression that the practice does not seem very concerned about their impact on the environment. She notices that computers are left on standby overnight and lights and radiators are left on all day, whether or not the consulting rooms are occupied. There is also a lot of waste – food from the practice lunches, paper that is shredded, and glass, cans and plastic are not recycled. There is a large car park, and Melanie also notes that the majority of staff drive to the practice, despite many living close by.

Melanie discusses her concerns with the practice manager over a practice lunch, who suggests that she help the practice formulate a 'Green Strategy'.

> **Exercise 10.3** *(Continued)* **Scenario**
> - How might Melanie evaluate how green the practice currently is?
> - How does the 'Green Strategy' fit in with other priorities of the practice? What are the drivers for adoption of her strategy?
> - What kinds of interventions might she suggest?
> - How can Melanie help to change the behaviour of the staff and patients of the practice?

Summary of issues

There are many different ways to change behaviours. For example, people can be incentivised to make certain choices. Incentives can be financial, rely on professional pressure and standing (such as publishing data) or can even be at an ethical or moral level. At the other end of the scale, people can be penalised from making the 'wrong' choices. People can be given information in a certain way to influence their choices. Alternatively, choice can be removed altogether and therefore people can be forced to take action. Checklists are very effective in certain situations to ensure that given activities have been completed.

In public health, the coalition government in the UK (elected into power in 2010) has put an emphasis on 'nudging' people to improve their health. In any situation, people will make choices by reflecting on conscious goals and values and by emotional and automatic reactions to environmental cues. Traditionally, those seeking to change behaviours (for example, in reducing obesity or stopping smoking) have focused on interventions that tap into the former cognitive system, providing examples of such goals and values. The 'nudge' theory says that to change behaviours, we must tap into the latter: *'the automatic, affective system that requires little or no cognitive engagement, being driven by immediate feelings and triggered by our environments'* (Marteau *et al.*, 2011). Melanie may wish to explore in her 'Green Strategy' how she could to 'nudge' people towards greener and more sustainable behaviours. For example, she may wish to give 'social norm' information about what other practices are doing, or she might make it easier for staff to make greener choices by placing a large recycling bin next to a small general bin in the practice kitchen.

Summary

Medical school is, in many ways, a fertile ground for developing leadership skills. The range of clinicians, settings and service users encountered mean that opportunities to learn from different ways of working – both good and bad – are abundant. The key to making the most of these experiences is to develop a critical eye and a desire to be involved. We have outlined many ways in which simple interactions can be used to explore, amongst other things, qualities in role models, information flows between members of the MDT and decision-making in theatre. On longer placements, medical students can develop their own improvement projects using PDSA cycles, can map out inefficiencies in patient care pathways and can help set the direction for a greener NHS. Although some of these latter suggestions may appear daunting for many students who see themselves as being the most junior of all clinical staff, the ability to persuade others that your contribution adds value is in and of itself an excellent leadership challenge. Once learned, this is likely lead to a more fulfilling career, and a much-improved NHS.

 Three things to try

1. Use the prompts in the opening chapter of this section to reflect on role models you have encountered through your placements. What values and qualities do they have that are important for providing high quality healthcare?
2. See if you can find an opportunity to shadow one of the clinicians or managers within your current department as they fulfil their management duties.
3. Ask a patient with a chronic condition if you can follow them down their 'journey' along a 'care pathway'. Note down their contacts with different members of the healthcare team across primary and secondary care. How do different team members communicate with eachother? What role does the patient have in this?

If you are a trainer, or have responsibility for teaching medical students on their clinical placements, how can you encourage students to think about the broader issues highlighted in this chapter and elsewhere in the book?

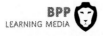

References

Darzi A (2008) *High Quality Care for All: NHS Next Stage Review final report* [Online] Available at www.dh.gov.uk/en/Publicationsandstatistics/ Publications/PublicationsPolicyAndGuidance/DH_085825 [Accessed 17/10/11].

Dharamshi R and Hillman T (2011) Going beyond audit. *BMJ Careers* [Online] Available at http://careers.bmj.com/careers/advice/view-article. html?id=20003642 [Accessed 17/10/11].

Dolan P *et al.* (2010) *MINDSPACE: influencing behaviour through public policy* [Online] Available at www.instituteforgovernment.org.uk/images/ files/MINDSPACE-full.pdf

Gawande A (2007) The Checklist. In *The New Yorker* [Online] Available at www.newyorker.com/reporting/2007/12/10/071210fa_fact_gawande [Accessed 17/10/11].

Green J and Britten B. Qualitative research and evidence based medicine. *BMJ* 1998; 316: 7139.

The Information Centre. *Quality and Outcomes Framework: Online GP practice results database* [Online] Available at www.qof.ic.nhs.uk [Accessed 17/10/11].

Institute for Healthcare Improvement. *Patient Safety: General.* [Online] Available at www.ihi.org/knowledge/Pages/Tools/WHO SurgicalSafetyChecklistGettingStarledkit.pdf [Accessed 17/10/11].

Janis IL (1982) *Groupthink: Psychological Studies of Policy Decisions and Fiascoes.* Boston, US: Houghton Mifflin.

Little P *et al.* Observational study of effect of patient centredness and positive approach on outcomes of general practice consultations. *BMJ* 2001; 323(7381): 908–911.

Marteau TM *et al.* Judging nudging: can nudging improve population health? *BMJ* 2011; 342: 228.

Michaels RK *et al.* Achieving the National Quality Forum's 'Never Events': Prevention of Wrong Site, Wrong Procedure, and Wrong Patient Operations. *Annals of Surgery* 2007; 245(4): 526–532.

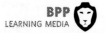

NHS Institute for Innovation and Improvement (2008) *Quality and Service Improvement Tools: Plan, Do, Study, Act (PDSA)* [Online] Available at www.institute.nhs.uk/quality_and_service_improvement_tools/quality_and_service_improvement_tools/plan_do_study_act.html [Accessed 17/10/11].

NHS Sustainable Development Unit (2010) *What can junior doctors do to improve health, save money and resources and reduce carbon pollution* [Online] Available at www.sdu.nhs.uk/documents/publications/Junior%20Docs.pdf [Accessed 17/10/11].

Paice E, Heard S and Moss F. How important are role models in making good doctors? *BMJ* 2002; 325(7366): 707.

Patel VM *et al*. What does leadership in surgery entail? *ANZ Journal of Surgery* 2010; 80: 876–883.

Snelgrove H, Gosling N and McAnulty G. The dissenting opinion: can simulation-based multi-professional training reduce 'groupthink'? *Postgrad Med J* [Online] Available at http://pmj.bmj.com/content/early/2011/01/21/pgmj.2010.109298.full.pdf [Accessed 17/10/11].

Thaler RH and Sunstein C (2008) *Nudge: improving decisions about health, wealth, and happiness*. Newhave, CT: Yale University Press.

Warren OJ and Carnall R. Medical leadership: why it's important, what is required, and how we develop it. *Postgrad Med J* 2011; 87: 27.

World Health Organization. *Safe Surgery Saves Lives* [Online] Available at www.who.int/patientsafety/safesurgery/en/ [Accessed 17/10/11].

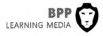

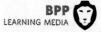

Chapter 11

Supporting Leadership Learning: Tutor Notes

Bob Klaber &
Lizzie Smith

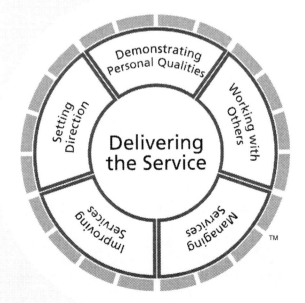

Chapter 11

Supporting Leadership Learning: Tutor Notes

 Chapter overview

This chapter focuses on how tutors and trainers can best support leadership learning, and explores a number of key concepts including:

- Ideas around work-based leadership learning
- The role of feedback in supporting learning
- Using the previous experiences of rotating trainees to improve care
- Moving beyond poor quality audit
- Focusing learning around quality improvement
- Pairing up clinicians and managers in peer-learning initiatives

Introduction

Previous chapters have focused on leadership learning in different clinical areas. While we hope the ideas discussed will provide useful material for anyone who is in a training or supervising role, the concepts, tools and techniques have been pitched at individual learners as they seek to develop their understanding and experience in leadership and management.

In this final chapter the emphasis changes to provide a tutor's or trainer's perspective on leadership development. Building on the individual ideas from the previous chapters, we will focus on broader concepts and organisational challenges with the aim of supporting trainers to develop work-based, experiential programmes of leadership learning within their workplace.

Work-based leadership learning

There are many definitions across the higher education literature around work-based learning, but within healthcare this can be boiled down to learning that is achieved as part of our work to provide care for patients. Leaders of medical education have championed for centuries the need for a significant proportion of a doctor's learning to be experiential or vocational. Since the full introduction of the European Working Time Directive (EWTD) within the NHS in 2009 (which reduced the average working week of junior doctors down to 48 hours per week) there has been huge debate on whether trainees gain sufficient experience of seeing patients, by the time they reach the end of their training period, to reach the standards required to become a consultant or GP. Professor Sir John Temple was asked by Medical Education England (MEE) to review the potential impact. In his report *Time for Training* (Temple, 2010) he is clear that high quality training *can* occur within the context of a 48-hour working week, although this is compromised where trainees have a major role in running out-of-hours services, have poor access to learning or are poorly supervised. Indeed, there may well be some specialties where, with a strong model of consultant teams and lifelong learning, postgraduate training programmes could, through higher quality and better focus, become shorter in duration.

It is somewhat odd that the medical profession is quick to staunchly defend every hour of clinical experience, yet until recent years there has been very little value placed on supporting doctors and medical students to develop skills in the key areas of leadership, management and education. With the introduction of the MLCF, and the response from statutory bodies and the Medical Royal Colleges to incorporating leadership and management competencies into medical curricula and guidance, there continues to be progress, although, for many, gaining these competencies is still perceived as a 'tick-box' exercise. A simple example of this comes at consultant interview. Why do so many interview panels accept a weekend leadership and management course, completed the month before the interview, as satisfactory 'management experience'? You can imagine a candidate trying to persuade a panel they were competent in a clinical procedure (endoscopy, for example) that had been taught for the first time on a two-day course the month before – they would be laughed out of the room, yet for leadership and management competencies this is the norm. Trainees should be exposed to work-based opportunities where they can experience leadership and management issues *throughout* their training, and the examples in this chapter will illustrate a number of ways this can be achieved. Changing this culture is key to driving forward real improvements in the years ahead.

Using feedback to support learning: providing insight

Perhaps the most important challenge for trainers to ensure high quality training is in developing the skills, techniques and mechanisms for all team members to receive thoughtful, developmental feedback. 'Developmental' means feedback that can be used by the person receiving it to change or improve some aspect of their work or behaviour. Jenny King, in her excellent work on the subject, relates feedback to providing insight:

> *Ultimately, feedback is about communication. The skills are generic: active listening; asking a balance of open, reflective, facilitating, and closed questions; challenging; and summarising. Giving feedback is not just to provide a judgment or evaluation. It is to provide insight. Without insight into their own strengths and limitations, trainees cannot progress or resolve difficulties. Thus, the key skills are to listen and ask, not, as is often the temptation, to tell and provide solutions.*

> (King, 1999)

This concept of insight or self-awareness is a crucial element of leadership, and plays a prominent part in the 'Developing Personal Qualities' domain of the MLCF. Using feedback to help learners develop insight and self-awareness is an extremely important area for trainers to work on.

Using feedback to support learning: Pendleton's 'rules'

Since the 1990s, driven in part by the development of well structured, standardised advanced life support courses, Pendleton's concepts have dominated feedback practice in healthcare in the UK (Pendleton *et al.*, 1984). Originally described with a focus on encouraging the person receiving feedback (the learner) to give their reflections on their own performance, and with an emphasis on placing positive comments alongside developmental feedback, these have fallen into a structure that are often referred to as 'Pendleton's rules':

1. The learner states what was done well.
2. The observer states what was done well.
3. The learner states what could be improved.

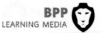

4.   The observer states what could be improved, and *how* this might be done

Pendleton's original work was very much conceptual rather than a set repertoire; the emergence of the word 'rules' has appeared subsequently. In many ways this has proved unhelpful as one of the major criticisms of this method of feedback is that it is too rigid, formulaic and predictable. Many learners get to know the pattern so well that there is a lack of meaningful discussion, and as much as the sections on 'what could be improved' are dressed up as being developmental, the common perception is 'this is the time for the negative criticism to come my way'.

As a result, although this method of feedback has helped considerably to move feedback on from being harsh and destructive, it rarely leads to genuine insight and actual change. Although it is clearly important to ensure the learner's view is gently obtained at some stage within the feedback conversation, launching into 'What did you do well?' a few seconds after the learner has heroically been leading a complex simulated resuscitation never seems to get anything more insightful than 'I remembered to start with ABC' or something similar.

Using feedback to support learning: other approaches

So, far from condemning Pendleton's ideas to the rubbish heap, how does one build on this idea of balancing feedback with strengths and areas for improvement, incorporating learner reflection and leaving the learner with a clear plan for how they can improve? Educationalists often refer to a 'narrative approach' where the learner and observer work together in a chronological way to recall and reflect on what happened step-by-step, teasing out learning points along the way. If well facilitated, this can be a very constructive approach and the observations and comments of other observers can be included to enrich the feedback. However, where the observation has been particularly long or complex it can be easy to get swamped in the detail of the beginning of the episode.

Silverman *et al.* describe a different approach that they have called 'agenda-led, outcomes based analysis' (Silverman *et al.*, 1996). In

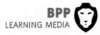

this method, as the observer, you start with the learners' agenda by asking them what problems they experienced and what help they would like from you and any other observers who might be present. You need to remain fully focused on the outcome the learner has chosen to achieve and not become distracted by other learning points you think are important. You do this by encouraging self-assessment and problem-solving before you, and eventually the whole group, contribute with problem-solving. Any feedback should be descriptive rather than judgmental and should also be balanced and objective as this will be most likely to effect change.

Without falling into the trap of giving the impression of there being such a thing as 'Klaber's feedback rules', the following guidance may help you reflect on your personal approach to giving feedback in a wide range of contexts:

- **Be learner-led:** ask the learner how they would most like to receive feedback; if they don't have particular views then give them two or three options which have worked well for others previously. Ensure the discussions are interactive and keep returning to the learner's self-perceptions and agenda.
- **Be flexible:** a successful facilitator/trainer will have several different techniques they feel comfortable using to deliver feedback. Being adaptable and responsive in real-time to whether or not different approaches are working is crucial.
- **Focus on achieving outcomes / improvement / change:** whatever strategies you adopt, it is important to focus on supporting the learner to continually seek improvement, however impressive their performance is. One of the definitions of excellence (in any walk of life) is a relentless desire to improve. Summarising with emphasis on outcomes and *how* to achieve improvements can be helpful.
- **Structure is important, but avoid being predictable:** much of the literature on feedback is focused on the importance of being structured, and while this is important, if the learner is only half-listening to the positive feedback as they wait for the imminent negatives, there is very little gained. This is a particular problem with the 'feedback sandwich' where positive feedback is positioned either side of an area for improvement.

- **Be descriptive, balanced and objective:** where possible, giving descriptive examples can help a learner to recall and reflect on particular issues. Being objective, balanced and focused on behaviours rather than becoming personal gives the process the feeling of being supportive and fair – it is extremely important for learners to feel positive about the feedback experience, even if there is much to work on, so that they can go on to effect change.

- **Take opportunities to feedback in different time frames:** although some learning opportunities are one-off episodes, ideally trainers should look to establish a strong relationship with learners where feedback can be given, and worked on, longitudinally in time. This approach is much more developmental and can offset that difficult dilemma, after observing a particularly problematic episode, about how much feedback one learner can receive in a single sitting.

- **Relate to principles, concepts and evidence:** if the opportunities arise, relating specific feedback points to wider concepts and evidence can be a useful way of contextualising them. This is also a helpful technique to depersonalise and broaden the ideas presented.

- **Don't hide from difficult feedback:** this is one area rarely mentioned in the feedback literature, despite being an area of significant concern for many trainers. As a trainer it can at times feel uncomfortable, vulnerable and risky contemplating highlighting problematic issues with a learner. In many ways this is a similar experience to how you approach difficult conversations with patients, where preparation is key. The ideas discussed above will help generate an approach that feels achievable. It is crucial that, at some point, appropriate feedback is given, as otherwise the learner will have no chance of gaining the insight needed to change.

'What can we learn from you?'

The section above describes a number of concepts concerning feedback, with a focus on the techniques trainers might adopt in giving feedback to trainees or students. Although all too rarely seen, there is great value in developing a feedback culture among peers (think about when you have seen regular feedback being given from consultant to consultant), and indeed *up* the traditional medical hierarchies. Multi-source or 360-degree feedback as described in Chapter 5 is one way of obtaining this, but does not need to be the only way – many of the ideas and techniques described above can work well in this situation if there is a culture of openness and active learning.

The idea of senior members of a team learning from junior colleagues on occasions is an important part of successful team dynamics, and is described in some detail in the section on flattened hierarchies in Chapter 4. This concept is worth considering from the very first day a new group of rotating doctors in training start in your department.

Although there are frustrations for long-term staff every time junior doctors rotate, there are aspects of these regular rotations that, if thoughtfully managed, can bring energy and innovation into the organisation. During their time as trainees, doctors in the UK move through many different departments and organisations to give them a breadth of experiences. It is these ideas and perspectives established senior clinicians should seek to learn from when a new group of trainees arrive at their department. The easiest way to achieve this is to run a session for the new doctors during their first week of work called *'What can we learn from you?'* Ideally, the session should be facilitated by one or two senior clinicians and a few managers, and run as an interactive small-group session. Ideas based on the trainees' experiences elsewhere can be brainstormed, captured and the potential for them to be adopted in your department discussed. This type of session can provide an excellent stimulus for trainees taking their own improvement projects forward. Additionally, our experience is that these sessions engender a considerable amount of enthusiasm and goodwill from trainees starting in our department. Although important for safe care, much of induction can feel like a 'mandatory telling-off' with long lists of things that must or cannot be done; this type of session is a helpful balance to that.

Moving beyond poor quality audit

Audit has formally been a part of healthcare in the UK since 1989, when the White Paper *Working Together for Patients* sought to

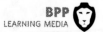

incorporate clinical audit into professional practice. Since then a huge amount of guidance about audit has been written (National Institute of Health and Clinical Excellence, 2002) and it has become a key part of postgraduate medical training in many countries across the world. Descriptions of audit, how it works and how it can improve care are given throughout this book. However, there is a problem with audit in the UK; too often it is of very poor quality and fails to moves beyond the data collection stage (Gnanalingham et al., 2001; John et al., 2004; Guryel et al., 2008). Even audit that is published in peer-reviewed articles can be of dubious quality (O'Gorman et al., 2007).

There has been varying guidance over the years from different Medical Royal Colleges in the UK about clinical audit. This has evolved into a perception, held by many educational supervisors, that 'every trainee must complete an audit in every post'. As a result, trainees on three-, four- and six-month placements often scramble around to find an audit they can take on. This is frequently given to them by a senior colleague, with variable explanation of the question underlying it. With the ensuing lack of ownership and the trainee's often unrealistic desire to complete the audit in a fixed time frame before they move on, it is of little surprise so few are completed and the learning is virtually nil (Hillman and Roueché, 2011). This creates a problem in that many trainees have never experienced a clinical audit that actually leads to improved care. While well intentioned, this approach to involving trainees in audit is often counter-productive and devalues the importance of clinical audit as a mainstay of clinical governance and high quality patient care.

Far from being eliminated, the new standards framework for health and social care in the UK (published by the Care Quality Commission in 2009); the requirement for Trust boards to publish 'Quality Accounts'; the need for providers to demonstrate they are achieving specific quality measures (CQuINs); as well as the plans for revalidation ensure that clinical audit is an important part of future healthcare. The challenge is to find ways in which trainees can contribute to, and learn from, clinical audit in a meaningful way. A starting point is moving away from an audit in *every* post. During their training, junior doctors should undoubtedly be involved in clinical audit; this should include developing a full understanding of the audit cycle and how it can drive improvement and change. This may mean working in teams, going back to a previous department to complete the work or contributing to a defined and focused part of a wider audit project. It is key to consider the potential improvements for patients and the potential learning for the trainee when planning any audit involving trainees.

If trainees are not completing an audit in every post then what should they be involved in alongside their clinical work? The answer has to come from the wider science of quality improvement – here the approach moves from scientific data collection to a more collaborative, investigative style that is focused on exploring problems, identifying solutions, and working as a team to improve patient care and experience. There are increasing numbers of resources that guide junior doctors through what quality improvement means in practice, and suggest how they can best be involved (Dharamshi and Hillman, 2011; Hillman and Roueché, 2011). The e-Learning for Healthcare (eLfH) leadership e-learning modules (called LeAD) also have a number of sessions focused on quality improvement. These can be accessed from www.e-lfh. org.uk/projects/lead/index.html. Although these resources may help individuals to participate in quality improvement work, the emphasis of this chapter is on how trainers can support leadership learning for the groups of junior doctors rotating through their department. The next section gives an example of one way in which this can be achieved.

Putting trainees at the heart of improving care

All departments have a wide range of ongoing leadership, management and quality improvement work. It makes a huge amount of sense to involve junior doctors in this work (Bethune *et al.*, 2011) both for their learning and also for the contributions that they can make to the work, yet it remains unusual for this to happen in a planned and systematic way. The aim has to be to open up all of the work of the department, and to encourage *all* junior doctors to contribute to at least one aspect of this. In the paediatric department at Imperial College Healthcare NHS Trust we have initiated a programme that attempts to do exactly that.

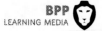

Case study: placing paediatric trainees at the heart of improving care for patients

Aim: to have a more co-ordinated approach to trainee involvement in the quality improvement, patient safety, management and governance work within the department:

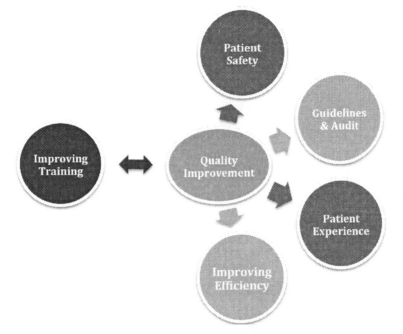

- All trainees are asked to participate in at least one of the six themes highlighted above during their time in the department. Each one has a theme lead (consultant).
- Each theme has a broad range of projects within it – these might be existing projects, or new projects based on ideas initiated by the trainee(s).
- Project outputs might be: presentations/improvement papers/teaching sessions/guidelines/reflective portfolio notes on personal learning.
- Each theme also has linked opportunities to attend and contribute to meetings, working groups and discussions within the department.

This programme is run every six months when the majority of the trainees rotate into the department. The starting point is a *'What can we learn from you?'* session as described earlier in this chapter, which runs in the junior doctors' first week. This is quickly followed up by a planning meeting where the trainees offer to contribute to different themes, and they are introduced to key supervisors,

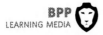

theme leads or project leads. They are also given information about associated meetings (eg risk management, quality and safety, patient user groups, coding, guidelines, training rep meetings, etc) that they will be invited to, and expected to contribute to, on the days they are in the department. Project work is supervised by individual project leads from across the consultant body, but the ethos of this involvement in the improvement work of the department is supported by monthly lunchtime meetings where trainees can update the training team how they are getting on. This monthly, informal discussion gives trainers/tutors the opportunity to encourage those trainees who are yet to become involved to do so, and to support and guide those who are already working on projects. The final meeting is focused on hearing about project outcomes and trainees' reflections on personal learning.

Working with, and learning from, managers

Another excellent way for trainees to gain work-based learning in aspects of leadership and management is to spend some time working with, and learning from, the managers in their department. As many organisations move towards working practices and structures where managers work closely alongside clinical leaders to plan and deliver care, this provides an outstanding opportunity for clinicians and managers to learn together through peer-learning initiatives.

With increasing evidence linking engagement between doctors and managers with improved organisational performance (Hamilton *et al.*, 2008; Spurgeon *et al.*, 2011), initiatives that bring doctors and managers together can contribute towards the improvement of healthcare services, in addition to providing valuable learning experiences. One example of this which has been shown to have significant benefits to patients and leads to powerful personal learning is called 'paired learning'. This initiative is based on using a 'buddy' approach, enabling trainees to gain insight into the world of management. This occurs through being paired with a manager in a way in which both can learn from each others' experience, while using their different areas of expertise to improve services for patients. Doctors and managers often approach healthcare

BPP
LEARNING MEDIA

issues from very different perspectives. The role of a junior doctor primarily involves applying medical knowledge and expertise to deliver care to individual patients. In contrast, healthcare management involves taking a broader view to ensure the necessary resources and processes are in place for the effective delivery of care. Pairing managers and doctors to learn about each others' roles and work on projects together can help trainees gain insight into how the wider resources and processes are agreed upon, and to understand who to approach to gain support for innovation and change. Likewise, managers can benefit through gaining insight into the way clinical decisions are made and the impact of clinical variation on the way services are organised.

Paired learning

The paired learning initiative at Imperial Healthcare NHS Trust brings together specialist registrar doctors with managers to learn through informal paired conversations, work shadowing, joint projects and workshops focused on leadership and improvement (Klaber *et al.*, 2011; Klaber and Lee, 2011).

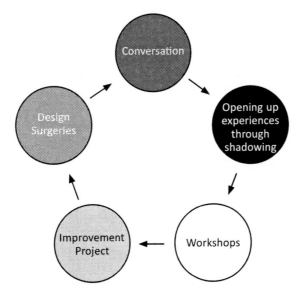

Figure 11.1 The paired learning initiative at Imperial Healthcare NHS Trust

The majority of leadership development programmes are not fully evaluated (Klaber *et al.*, 2009) and therefore omit a step which is crucial for understanding the impact of interventions and justifying the use of resources. Paired learning has been piloted and evaluated in detail; the qualitative analysis suggests that the following points should be considered when designing and running a manager-clinician peer-learning programme:

Leadership and role-modelling: paired learning was initiated by a team of senior managers and clinicians who could speak from personal experience of the benefits of collaboration, as well as provide access to a network of potential clinical and management participants. It is worth bearing in mind that while there are fantastic examples of successful partnership working between managers and doctors in the NHS, there are many areas in which negative and unhelpful perceptions of non-clinical management persist. It is likely that some trainees will have been exposed to such attitudes early in their careers, and so may benefit from being exposed to the leadership of a senior clinician who is a role model for strong partnership working with the management team.

Participants: there is a strong case for co-developing doctors and managers early in their training so they can build on this collaborative approach throughout their careers. The paired learning pilot programme worked well with doctors at specialist registrar level (ST3–8), who are starting to consider the leadership responsibilities they will encounter as a consultant. There are undoubtedly possibilities for starting these types of initiatives at the beginning of training by involving foundation year doctors, and organisations may want to encourage newly appointed consultants to participate in similar schemes. The managers in the pilot were mainly service or general managers (Bands 7–8), but there is no reason that others (eg from a finance, performance or information background) could not get involved. Schemes may also want to take a multiprofessional approach through involving allied health professionals in small learning groups. There is also the opportunity to run these groups and projects across traditional organisational boundaries (eg across primary and secondary care).

Establishing pairs: doctors and managers can be paired up in a number of ways. Findings from the paired learning pilot align

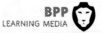

with the evidence for successful mentoring processes where a likely personality 'fit' increases the chance of a successful relationship (Clutterbuck and Ragins, 2002). Participants should be given the opportunity to get to know each other informally before choosing to work together, although some may prefer to be allocated a 'buddy'. Pairing individuals from within a department works well where individuals wish to focus on a specific work-based project or specialty, while pairings across different departments can help facilitate the sharing of knowledge and innovation across divisions and specialties.

Designing the programme: the paired learning pilot incorporated five different learning components, although it would be perfectly possible to establish a programme that focused on only two or three of these.

Conversation: in the paired learning pilot, both doctors and managers identified learning about the other person's experience through paired conversations as the most useful component of the programme. Pairs commonly used these informal discussions to learn about their respective professional hierarchies, the processes involved in decision-making, and the different language used by managers and doctors. Pairing individuals who are at broadly similar stages in their career can avoid either participant from feeling intimidated or unable to ask 'the silly question'. For specialist registrars the opportunity to learn about management in an offline environment is invaluable, and can increase confidence and preparedness for their future involvement in management activities.

Opening up experiences through shadowing: pairs might also spend time shadowing each other. This is a good opportunity for trainees to gain firsthand experience of management activities and to contribute to strategic and operational meetings. Trainees should be encouraged to feed their clinical perspective into management meetings. They may find they can shed light on longstanding issues and help develop robust plans for service improvement.

Workshops: facilitated workshops where a group of doctors and managers learn alongside each other can be helpful. Although the two groups have different learning needs, sessions based on developing the skills and behaviours to lead change are a useful approach (eg developing self-awareness and a shared purpose; understanding the NHS context; developing skills and tools for change; and designing services for safety and quality).

Improvement projects and design surgeries: pairs may also be encouraged to work on a shared improvement project or provide a different perspective on each other's projects. These projects can be self-led, allocated or chosen from a menu of projects that the organisation is keen to run. Project leads should put aside time to provide coaching support or technical expertise through 'design surgeries' to help projects achieve their outcomes and maximise learning.

Finally, pairs should be encouraged to feedback their experiences to colleagues both within the paired learning cohort and within their department or other forums in the organisation. Throughout, trainees should be supported to build long term connections that they rely on for support or advice in the future.

Further information on the the paired learning pilot can be found at www.imperial.nhs.uk/pairedlearning and in the references below.

Summary

The quality of education and training junior doctors and medical students receive is hugely dependent upon the presence of outstanding, dynamic and committed tutors to facilitate their learning. This chapter has focused on providing tutors and trainers with ideas on how they can initiate, and develop, high quality work-based learning programmes that will support their trainees to develop leadership and management experience and capabilities. We have reviewed and challenged traditional models of feedback, explored a few of the issues concerning how trainees encounter clinical audit and examined how trainees might get involved with quality improvement work within their department. Finally, through illustrating the paired learning programme, we have demonstrated the value of developing opportunities for peer learning between managers and clinicians.

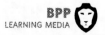

Three things to try

1. Think about how you usually give junior trainees feedback. Are there are any aspects of what you do that could be done differently to better support learning?
2. Think about how you might facilitate each group of new trainees who rotate into your department in actively contributing to the ongoing quality and safety work.
3. Think about how different people within your department or organisation might be able to pair up in a peer-learning environment, where they can learn through conversation, shadowing and working on a project together.

References and further reading

Bethune R, Roueché A and Hilman T. Is quality of care improving? Improvement efforts need to be targeted at junior doctors. *BMJ (Clinical Research Ed.)* 2011; 342, p.d1323.

Clutterbuck D and Ragins B (2002) *Designing and Sustaining a Mentoring Programme, Mentoring and Diversity: an international perspective.* Melbourne: Butterworth-Heinemann.

Dharamshi R and Hillman T. Going beyond audit. *BMJ Careers.* [Online] Available at: http://careers.bmj.com/careers/advice/view-article.html?id=20003642 [Accessed 17/10/11].

Gnanalingham J, Gnanalingham MG and Gnanalingham KK. An audit of audits: are we completing the cycle? *Journal of the Royal Society of Medicine* 2001; 94(6): pp. 288–289.

Guryel E, Acton, K and Patel S. Auditing orthopaedic audit. *Annals of the Royal College of Surgeons of England* 2008; 90(8): pp. 675–678.

Hamilton P. *et al.* (2008). *Engaging Doctors: Can Doctors Influence Organisational Performance?* Coventry, UK: NHS Institute for Innovation and Improvement.

Hillman T and Roueché A (2011) Quality Improvement. *BMJ Careers.* [Online] Available at: http://careers.bmj.com/careers/advice/view-article.html?id=20002524 [Accessed 17/10/11].

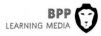

Hillman T and Roueché A. Quality Improvement. *BMJ Careers* [Online] Available at: http://careers.bmj.com/careers/advice/view-article. html?id=20002524 [Accessed 17/10/11].

John CM, Mathew DE and Gnanalingham MG. An audit of paediatric audits. *Archives of Disease in Childhood* 2004; 89(12): pp. 1128–1129.

King J. Giving feedback. *BMJ* 1999; 318(7200): p. 2.

Klaber RE *et al.* A structured approach to planning a work-based leadership development programme for doctors in training. *The International Journal of Clinical Leadership* 2009; 16(3): pp. 121–129.

Klaber RE *et al.* How pairing clinicians with managers could speed up clinical excellence. *Health Service Journal* 2011 (20 September).

Klaber RE and Lee J. Clinical Leadership and Management in the NHS: Paired learning. *J R Soc Med* 2011; 104: 436.

National Institute of Clinical Excellence (2002) *Principles of Best Practice in Clinical Audit.* London: NICE.

O'Gorman CS, Ziedan Y and O'Neill MB. An evaluation of Medline published paediatric audits from 1966 to 1999. *Archives of Disease in Childhood* 2007; 92(4): pp. 309–311.

Pendleton D *et al.* (1984) *The consultation: an approach to learning and teaching.* Oxford: Oxford University Press.

Silverman J, Krurtz S and Draper J. The Calgary-Cambridge approach to communication skills teaching. Agenda-led, outcome-based analysis of the consultation. *Educ Gen Prac* 1996; 7: pp. 288–299.

Spurgeon P, Mazelan PM and Barwell F. Medical engagement: a crucial underpinning to organizational performance. *Health Serv Manage Res* 2011; 24(3): pp. 114–120.

Temple, J. *Time for Training,* Medical Education England [Online] Available at www.mee.nhs.uk/PDF/14274%20Bookmark%20Web%20Version.pdf [Accessed 17/10/11].

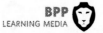

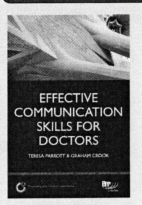

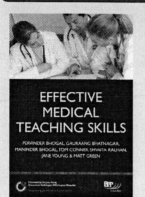

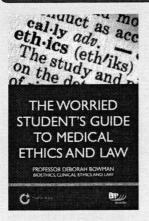

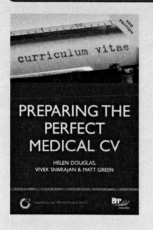

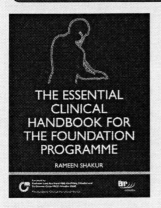

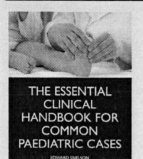